AF324185

PARKINSON'S DEMENTIA

Edited by Clive Ballard MD

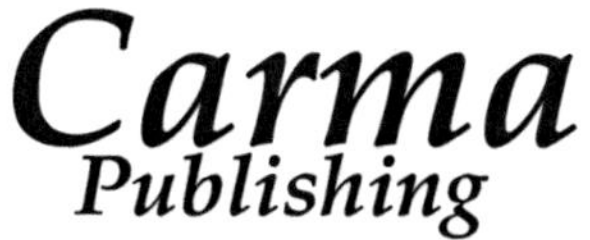

Carma Publishing

Published by Carma Publishing LLC, Delray Beach, Florida, USA

Orders may be placed through the website www.carmapubs.com

ISBN: 978-0-9769581-9-2
0-9769581-9-8

Printed in the United States of America

Foreword

Parkinson's Dementia edited by Clive Ballard MD is one of a set of books planned to be published in 2007 covering the dementing diseases including, initially, Alzheimer's, Parkinson's, Huntington's, and Other Dementias. Developments in Frontotemporal and Vascular Dementia are moving at such a pace that books on these topics will be published at a later date.

In this age of the Internet, we have used the available technologies to publish both in print and on the Carma Publishing website www.carmapubs.com. The book editors and the authors of the individual articles will be monitoring the developments in their areas of expertise and will be updating their articles to reflect the advances in our understanding of the diagnosis, treatment, etiology, pathophysiology, and management of these diseases so that the articles will always be up to date. The updated articles will be published on the www.carmapubs.com website within days of the article being accepted by the book editor so that readers and libraries can expect that they will always have the most up-to-date information available anywhere. The print versions (books) will be updated from time to time.

Access to the online articles is password protected and passwords are distributed by Carma Publishing to customer e-mail addresses either when they order online at www.carmapubs.com or by completing the form in this book and sending it to Carma Publishing with proof of purchase.

We thank Dr. Howard Feldman for his guidance in publishing these books.

Password Request Form

To receive a password to the articles and all updates online for 12 months from the date of purchase, complete this form and send it to Carma Publishing with proof of purchase.

By Fax: 561-279-0384
By e-mail: service@carmapubs.com

We remind our customers that your password is for your personal access to these articles and may not be shared with others. Protect your password at all times. Abuse will result in cancellation of your password.
Licenses are available for group and site use.
Contact Us by e-mail: <u>service@carmapubs.com</u>.

Please print legibly or type.
All fields must be completed.

Name: ____

Street Address: _______________________________________

City: __________________ State/Province: ________________

Zip/Postal Code: ______________ Country: _______________

Organization/Company: _________________________________

Department: ____

Telephone: ___________________________________

E-mail: _____________________________________

Proof of purchase must accompany the form.

Contents

Related Titles

Alzheimer's Dementia edited by Rachelle S. Doody

Huntington's Dementia edited by Blair Leavitt

Other Dementias edited by David Geldmacher

Alzheimer's Essentials by Bretten C. Gordeau & Jeffrey Hillier

www.carmapubs.com

1

Dementia with Lewy Bodies

Clive Ballard

Address correspondence to Dr. Clive Ballard, Wolfson Centre for Age-Related Diseases, Wolfson Building, Hodgkin Building, Guy's Campus, King's College London, London, SE1 1UL, UK.
E-mail: Clive.ballard@kcl.ac.uk

OUTLINE

INTRODUCTION

Dementia with Lewy bodies (DLB) was first reported in the 1960s[1]. Subsequently, several small case series emerged, largely from Japan, in the 1970s and early 1980s[2], before reports describing larger groups of patients in the late 1980s and early 1990s[3–7] began to highlight the frequency of the syndrome and the characteristic clinical features. It was not, however, until the emergence of ubiquitin staining and the later identification of α-synuclein as the fundamental core pathological hallmark that the true extent of the pathology and importance of the syndrome was acknowledged.

PREVALENCE

Dementias associated with cortical Lewy bodies are traditionally classified as DLB or Parkinson's disease dementia (PDD). DLB is characterized by visual hallucinations, fluctuating cognition, and motor parkinsonism arising concurrently with or after the onset of dementia[8]. PDD is diagnosed when dementia ensues 1 year or more after the onset of Parkinson's disease. DLB accounts for about 20% of late-onset dementia cases[8], implying an approximate prevalence of 1% in people over the age of 65. Dementia eventually develops in the majority of older patients with a diagnosis of Parkinson's disease[9], with an estimated cross-sectional community prevalence of PDD of 0.5% in people over the age of 65[10].

PROFILE OF COGNITIVE DEFICITS

The cognitive profile of both PDD and DLB has been characterized as a visuospatial, attentional, and executive impairment with relatively less memory impairment[8,11]. This is based on studies comparing DLB and PDD patients to patients with Alzheimer's disease. The overall profile of cognitive deficits is similar in the two syndromes, with both PDD and DLB patients exhibiting significantly more marked executive and less memory deficits than patients with Alzheimer's disease. Interestingly, fluctuating attention, a key feature of DLB, is evident in both DLB and PDD, but not in Alzheimer's disease or Parkinson's disease without dementia, and less marked fluctuation of attention was also found in DLB patients without parkinsonism[12]. An additional study comparing pentagon copying in patients with DLB and PDD suggested a similar severity of impairment in the two conditions and a pattern of errors indicating executive dysfunction[13]. A further study, although suggesting marked executive dysfunction in both PDD and DLB, illustrated that in the context of mild dementia, patients with DLB had a significantly lower score on the Dementia Rating Scale Conceptualization subscale than patients with Parkinson's disease, suggesting that executive impairment is more pronounced in patients with DLB than in patients with Parkinson's disease with mild dementia[14]. Overall, however, the profile of cognitive impairments in DLB and PDD appears to be similar and distinct from Alzheimer's disease.

NEUROPSYCHIATRIC SYMPTOMS

Psychiatric symptoms are common in all dementia syndromes, but a characteristic psychiatric profile has been reported in patients with DLB and PDD. Visual hallucinations and delusions are much more common in DLB than in Alzheimer's disease, occurring in 60–70% of patients with DLB[15,16], whereas in PDD, hallucinations (45–50%), but not delusions (15–24%), were more common than in Alzheimer's disease[16,17]. REM sleep behavior disorders are also substantially more common in DLB and PDD than in other dementias, and may actually precede the dementia syndrome in many patients[18]. Depression, apathy, and anxiety are common in most dementias, but probably have a higher frequency in DLB[15,16] and PDD[9], consistent with the high frequency of depression found in Parkinson's disease[19].

DIAGNOSIS

International, operationalized, clinical criteria for the diagnosis of DLB were agreed at a consensus conference in 1995 and published the following year[8]. These criteria highlighted three core diagnostic features: fluctuating cognition, persistent or recurrent visual hallucinations, and spontaneous parkinsonism; two of which had to be present in the context of a dementia syndrome to support a diagnosis of probable DLB. In addition, an arbitrary 1-year rule was applied to distinguish DLB from PDD, and a diagnosis of DLB was prohibited in people with more than a 1-year history of Parkinson's disease prior to dementia. Autopsy validation studies indicate that although specificity of diagnosis is generally good (80%), the sensitivity of these criteria for DLB may be as low as 50% in some studies. Aided by emerging scientific data, the International DLB Consortium has, therefore, recently revised the criteria originally proposed for the clinical and pathological diagnosis of DLB[20], and the role of special investigations was reviewed. Additional clinical features (REM sleep behavior disorder and severe neuroleptic sensitivity) and functional imaging changes (dopamine transporter scan or myocardial scintigraphy) are now considered to be suggestive of DLB, and a diagnosis of probable DLB can now be made in the presence of one core feature, if one or more suggestive features are also present. In addition, more detailed descriptions are provided to assist clinicians in identifying the core features appropriately. Given the recent availability of these criteria, they have not yet been validated prospectively.

Diagnostic criteria have not yet been formerly developed for PDD, although an international consortium is currently addressing this issue. By default, however, as a consequence of the DLB criteria, PDD can only be diagnosed in people with more than 1 year of parkinsonism prior to the onset of dementia. Most clinical studies in the area suggest that PDD patients have a similar profile of clinical symptoms to those with DLB and that more than 90% of PDD patients meet the diagnostic criteria for DLB apart from the 1-year rule. No criteria have been developed or validated based on these principles.

Three pivotal autopsy studies[21,22,23], including more than 100 patients with Parkinson's disease who developed dementia, clearly demonstrated that identifying a group of patients with Parkinson's disease who subsequently develop dementia (diagnosed using DSMIII or DSMIIIR criteria for generic dementia) predicts a characteristic neuropathological picture at autopsy characterized by widespread cortical Lewy body pathology. Only 6% of these patients had sufficient plaque and tangle pathology to meet current diagnostic criteria for Alzheimer's disease, and the severity of cognitive deficits was predominantly associated with the severity of cortical Lewy body pathology. This would indicate that a simple approach to diagnosis based on the presence of Parkinson's disease and the subsequent development of dementia is sufficient to diagnose PDD accurately, and that more complex criteria may be unnecessary.

SUMMARY

DLB and PDD are common dementia syndromes, with characteristic and distressing symptom profiles that enable accurate diagnosis. Further contributions to this section of this book will highlight key emerging issues pertaining to the neuropathological and neurochemical basis of the syndrome and related symptoms, the underlying disease mechanisms, the importance of understanding the genetic contribution, and will provide an overview to inform clinical management.

REFERENCES

1.   Woodard JS. Concentric hyaline inclusion body formation in mental disease analysis of twenty-seven cases. J Neuropathol Exp Neurol. 1962;21:442-9.
2.   Kosaka K, Yoshimura M, Ikeda K, et al. Diffuse type of Lewy body disease: progressive dementia with abundant cortical Lewy bodies and senile changes of varying degree-a new disease? Clin Neuropathol. 1984;3:185-92.
3.   Gibb WR, Luthert PJ, Janota I, et al. Cortical Lewy body dementia: clinical features and classification. J Neurol Neurosurg Psychiatry. 1989;52:185-92.
4.   Byrne EJ, Lennox G, Lowe J, et al. Diffuse Lewy body disease: clinical features in 15 cases. J Neurol Neurosurg Psychiatry. 1989;52:709-17.
5.   Hansen L, Salmon D, Galasko D, et al. The Lewy body variant of Alzheimer's disease: a clinical and pathological entity. Neurology. 1990;40:1-8.

6.	Perry RH, Irving D, Blessed G, Fairbairn A, Perry EK. Senile dementia of Lewy body type. A clinically and neuropathologically distinct form of Lewy body dementia in the elderly. J Neurol Sci. 1990;95:119-39.

7.	McKeith IG, Perry RH, Fairbairn AF, Jabeen S, Perry EK. Operational criteria for senile dementia of Lewy body type (SDLT). Psychol Med. 1992;22:911-22.

8.	McKeith IG, Galasko D, Kosaka K, Perry EK, Dickson DW, Hansen LA, Salmon DP, Lowe J, Mirra SS, Byrne EJ, Lennox G, Quinn NP, Edwardson JA, Ince PG, Bergeron C, Burns A, Miller BL, Lovestone S, Collerton D, Jansen EN, Ballard C, de Vos RA, Wilcock GK, Jellinger KA, Perry RH. Consensus guidelines for the clinical and pathologic diagnosis of dementia with Lewy bodies (DLB): report of the consortium on DLB international workshop. Neurology. 1996;47:1113-24.

9.	Aarsland D, Andersen K, et al. Prevalence and characteristics of dementia in Parkinson disease - an 8-year prospective study. Arch Neurol. 2003;60:387-92.

10.	Aarsland D, Zaccai J, Brayne C. A systematic review of prevalence studies of dementia in Parkinson's disease. Mov Disord. 2005;20:1255-63.

11.	Pillon B, Boller F, Levy R, et al. Cognitive deficits and dementia in Parkinson's disease. Handbook of Neuropsychology, 2nd ed. Amsterdam: Elsevier Sciences BV; 2001:311-71.

12.	Ballard CG, Aarsland D, et al. Fluctuations in attention - PD dementia vs DLB with parkinsonism. Neurology. 2002;59:1714-20.

13.	Cormack F, Aarsland D, Ballard C, et al. Pentagon drawing and neuropsychological performance in Dementia with Lewy Bodies, Alzheimer's disease, Parkinson's disease and Parkinson's disease with dementia. Int J Geriatr Psychiatry. 2004;19:371-7.

14.	Aarsland D, Litvan I, Salmon D, et al. Performance on the dementia rating scale in Parkinson's disease with dementia and dementia with Lewy bodies: comparison with progressive supranuclear palsy and Alzheimer's disease. J Neurol Neurosurg Psychiatry. 2003;74:1215-20.

15.	Ballard C, Holmes C, McKeith I, et al. Psychiatric morbidity in dementia with Lewy bodies: a prospective clinical and neuropathological comparative study with Alzheimer's disease. Am J Psychol. 1999;156:1039-45.

16.	Klatka L, Louis E, Schiffer RB. Psychiatric features in diffuse Lewy body disease; a clinicopathologic study using Alzheimer's disease and Parkinson's disease control groups. Neurology. 1996;47:1148-52.

17.   Aarsland D, Cummings JL, Larsen JP. Neuropsychiatric differences between Parkinson's disease with dementia and Alzheimer's disease. Int J Geriatr Psychiatry. 2001;16(2):184-91,.

18.   Ferman TJ, Boeve BF, Ivnik RJ, et al. DLB fluctuations: specific features that reliably differentiate from AD and normal aging. Neurology. 2004;62:181-7.

19.   Tandberg E, Larsen JP, Aarsland D, et al. Risk factors for depression in Parkinson disease. Arch Neurol. 1997;54:625-30.

20.   McKeith IG, Dickson DW, Lowe J, et al. Consortium on DLB. Diagnosis and management of dementia with Lewy bodies: third report of the DLB Consortium. Neurology. 2005;65:1863-72.

21.   Aarsland D, Perry R, Brown A, et al. Neuropathology of dementia in Parkinson's disease: a prospective, community-based study. Ann Neurol. 2005;58:773-6.

22.   Apaydin H, Ahlskog JE, Parisi JE, et al. Parkinson's disease neuropathology: later-developing dementia and loss of the levo-dopa response. Arch Neurol. 2002;59:102-12.

23.   Braak H, Del Tredici K, Rub U, et al. Staging of brain pathology related to sporadic Parkinson's disease. Neurobiol Aging. 2003;24:197-211.

2

Neuropathology and Neurochemistry of Dementia with Lewy Bodies and Parkinson's Disease Dementia

Martin Broadstock[1], Elaine K. Perry[1,2], Robert Perry[2], and Paul T. Francis[1]

[1]Wolfson Centre for Age-Related Diseases, King's College London, London, UK;
[2]IAH Research Laboratories, Institute for Ageing and Health, University of Newcastle upon Tyne, Newcastle upon Tyne, UK.

Address correspondence to Dr. Martin Broadstock, Wolfson Centre for Age-Related Diseases, Guy's Campus, King's College London, St Thomas Street, London SE1 1UL, UK.
E-mail: martin.broadstock@kcl.ac.uk

OUTLINE

Introduction
Cortical Changes in DLB and PPD
Cholinergic Neurotransmission
Glutaminergic Neurotransmission
Dopaminergic Neurotransmission
Other Neurotransmitter Systems
References

INTRODUCTION

Over 30 years ago, an intensive effort was undertaken to understand the neurochemistry and neuropathological changes in dementia, exemplified by the debilitating disorder Alzheimer's disease. The results of such studies led to the development of rational treatment strategies that continue to benefit patients. However, as studies became more sophisticated and clinicians rediscovered an interest in dementia because of the potential for symptomatic treatment, it became clear that there are several different neurodegenerative conditions that give rise to dementia syndromes and that each has distinct neurochemical pathology[1,2]. This has important treatment implications since what works for one may not work for another or, at the extreme, may exacerbate existing symptoms. It is, therefore, apparent that a detailed understanding of the neurotransmitter function in each condition is not merely academic, but could lead to rational drug design and treatment strategies appropriate for that group of patients. Dementia with Lewy bodies (DLB) has clinicopathological features that overlap with either Alzheimer's disease or Parkinson's disease, as well as features that help to distinguish it, including fluctuations in cognitive impairment and a higher prevalence of visual hallucinations. Similarly, Parkinson's disease with dementia (PDD) retains the motor complications associated with Parkinson's disease, with the additional impairment of dementia. On this basis, it would be expected that the neurochemistry and neuropathology of DLB and PDD would have some similarities with both Alzheimer's disease and Parkinson's disease.

CORTICAL CHANGES IN DLB AND PDD

The main correlates of cognitive impairment in Alzheimer's disease are cortical atrophy due to the loss of pyramidal neurons and their associated synapses, tangles within pyramidal neurons, and cholinergic dysfunction[2,3]. In Alzheimer's disease, gross atrophy can be observed in the medial temporal, frontal, and parietal lobes. However, in the lesser-studied areas of DLB and PDD, there are a number of inconsistencies between studies related to cortical changes. Magnetic resonance imaging studies investigating hippocampal atrophy have suggested that loss of hippocampal neurons in PDD is similar or even greater than that observed in Alzheimer's disease[4,5]. However, a further study suggests that such hippocampal loss is actually greater in Alzheimer's disease compared to PDD. This same study reported a loss of gray matter volume in frontal, temporal, parietal, and occipital areas in PDD compared to controls[6]. A more recent study found significantly higher rates of brain atrophy using serial magnetic resonance imaging in PDD of 1.12 ± 0.98%/year, and compared to cognitively intact Parkinson's disease patients (0.31 ± 0.69%/year) and control subjects (0.34 ± 0.76%/year)[7]. If cortical atrophy does indeed occur in PDD, one might expect this to be the substrate of dementia, yet interestingly, no correlations were observed between increased atrophy rates and Mini-Mental State Examination scores.

Many reports show that Alzheimer's disease pathology, evidenced by senile plaques and tangles, does occur in PDD/DLB to a greater extent than Parkinson's disease, but at a level insufficient to diagnose concurrent Alzheimer's disease[8]. Therefore, these neuropathological correlates of dementia are unlikely to underlie the cognitive decline observed in these cases. Furthermore, there is little evidence of extensive loss of cortical synapses (determined by synaptophysin immunoreactivity) in DLB in the absence of concurrent Alzheimer's disease[9].

The extent of cortical Lewy body pathology is now considered an important determinant of cognitive impairment in both DLB and PDD, with widespread diffuse or transitional Lewy bodies in 97% of cases in a recent study[8], in comparison with the relatively few in Parkinson's disease without dementia.

CHOLINERGIC NEUROTRANSMISSION

The status of the cholinergic system in Alzheimer's disease, PDD, and DLB is summarized in Figure 1. In comparison with both Alzheimer's disease and Parkinson's disease, there is an increased loss of both cholinergic neurons and choline acetyltransferase (ChAT) activity in

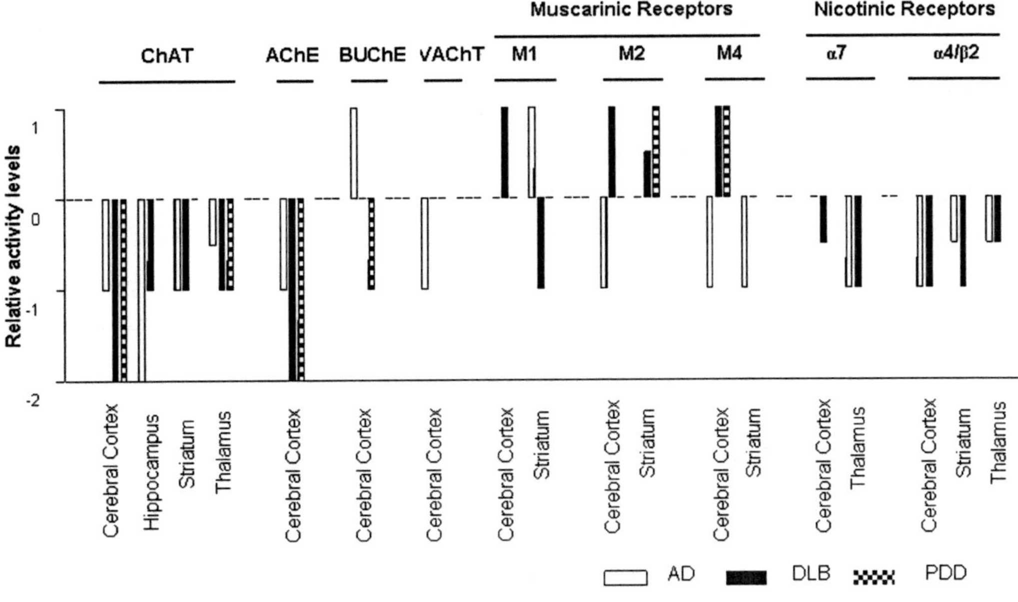

FIGURE 1.

both PDD and DLB, especially within the cerebral cortex. These reductions in presynaptic cholinergic neuronal activities are not only of a greater magnitude, but also become apparent earlier in disease progression compared to Alzheimer's disease[10–12]. One difference between DLB and Alzheimer's disease is the additional loss of neurons in DLB within the cholinergic components of the basal ganglia nuclei, the caudate-putamen (striatum), and the pedunculopontine nucleus.

Interestingly, both ChAT deficits and increased muscarinic M2 and M4 receptor binding are apparent in some regions of the temporal cortex of DLB patients with visual hallucinations compared to those without[10,11,13]. Regarding ChAT deficits, the greatest differences were seen in areas of the temporal cortex involved with visual recognition (Brodmann's area [BA] 36) versus the parietal cortex, which is involved with the representation of visual objects in space and the interpretation of visual input into appropriate motor activity[14]. In this study, many of the DLB patients who were experiencing visual hallucinations were being treated with levodopa, which is known to induce visual hallucinations in some patients with DLB and PDD. An imbalance in cholinergic and dopaminergic activity may exacerbate or precipitate hallucinations in these patients[11]. It has been suggested that the striatal cholinergic deficiency may contribute to the lesser degree of extrapyramidal symptoms seen in DLB compared to Parkinson's disease, which retains normal striatal cholinergic activity. However, this has not yet been supported by clinical-pathological correlations, and it is likely that less-extensive substantia nigra neuronal loss may also be responsible. The decreased thalamic cholinergic activity is probably reflective of the loss of pedunculopontine nuclei, which undoubtedly occurs similarly in DLB as in Parkinson's disease[15]. Whether this relates to attentional dysfunction and/or disturbances in consciousness, which are more extensive in DLB compared to Alzheimer's disease, remains to be established.

In two studies, M1 receptors were preserved or up-regulated in the temporal cortex in DLB compared to Alzheimer's disease, but appeared to be reduced in the hippocampus in both DLB and Alzheimer's disease[14,16,17]. Furthermore, there is some evidence of the uncoupling of M1 receptors from their intracellular cascade in Alzheimer's disease. Preservation of M1 receptor number and function in the temporal cortex in DLB may partially explain why patients with DLB have a particularly beneficial response to cholinergic agents, such as acetylcholinesterase (ACh) inhibitors[18].

Increased M2 receptor binding in the inferior cingulate cortex and the superior BA 32 is seen in DLB compared to controls, and DLB with either visual hallucinations or delusions compared to DLB without. These findings may reflect a compensatory mechanism for preserving ACh on those surviving cholinergic neurons. M2 receptors are presynaptic, inhibitory, G-protein coupled receptors, whose activation serves to reduce further ACh (and other neurotransmitters) release. In the same study, an increase in M4 receptor binding was observed in the superior cingulate cortex of DLB patients with impaired consciousness compared to those without, and increased binding in superior BA 32 of those DLB patients with visual hallucinations compared to those without[13].

Nicotine binding is significantly reduced in the substantia nigra in both Parkinson's disease and DLB[19], however, neuronal loss accounts for much of the nicotinic receptor loss in Parkinson's disease, but not in DLB. Parkinson's disease and DLB patients had neuronal losses of 70 and 40%, respectively, while nicotine binding was reduced by 70% in both diseases. This suggests that, similar to other parts of the brain, loss of cholinergic function in the substantia nigra precedes the degeneration and loss of neurons in DLB.

High-affinity nicotinic receptor loss has also been investigated in the temporal cortex in both DLB and Alzheimer's disease[19,20]. In Alzheimer's disease, the loss of nicotinic receptors within this region mirrors the loss of ChAT and ACh. However, in DLB, the nicotinic receptor loss was not as extensive as that observed in Alzheimer's disease, despite the greater reduction of ChAT in patients with DLB compared to those with Alzheimer's disease. These results suggest alternative mechanisms for nicotinic receptor loss, rather than receptor loss as a consequence of loss of cholinergic neurons. Interestingly, the area of highest Lewy body density in the parahippocampal gyrus did not correlate with the greatest nicotinic receptor loss in DLB; in fact, nicotinic receptor levels were actually higher in this region in DLB. More relevant to the symptoms of memory loss that occur in both Alzheimer's disease and DLB patients may be the significant receptor loss in the dentate granular area. Alzheimer's disease patients also have reduced projections from the entorhinal cortex to the dentate granular area, which may account for the more severe memory deficits seen in Alzheimer's disease patients compared to those with DLB.

In DLB, nicotinic receptor changes in the cortex include a loss of the high-affinity agonist binding site (reflecting the $\alpha4\beta2$ subtype)[21], but no consistently reported change in the $\alpha7$ subunit or α-bungarotoxin binding site. These observations are reversed in the thalamus where there is little change in nicotine binding, but a highly significant reduction in α-bungarotoxin binding in the reticular nucleus. Similar nicotinic receptor abnormalities occur in Alzheimer's disease and, insofar as have been investigated, in Parkinson's disease. For example, within the striatum, there is a greater loss of nicotine binding in

Parkinson's disease than in DLB[22]. This observation is consistent with the extensive loss of dopaminergic afferents in the basal ganglia in Parkinson's disease compared to DLB. However, this loss of α6/α3 nicotinic receptors in DLB is still significantly greater compared to control cases[23].

Nicotinic receptors of the α7 subtype are reduced in DLB compared to Alzheimer's disease or controls[21,24]. This could have significance for DLB, since α7 nicotinic receptors are thought to have a role in the release of the neurotransmitter glutamate. Deficiencies in α7 nicotinic receptors may also affect hallucinations in patients with DLB. In a study of DLB patients who either did or did not experience hallucinations, only those who experienced hallucinations had a deficiency in α7 nicotinic receptors in the temporal cortex in areas associated with encoding complex recognition (BA 20 and 36)[25]. There were no significant differences in high-affinity nicotinic receptors for DLB patients who experienced hallucinations versus those who did not. However, this study and another study[20] showed that there were significant differences in high-affinity nicotinic receptor levels between DLB and age-matched controls. In contrast, high-affinity nicotinic receptor binding in the temporal cortex (BA 20 and 36) served to differentiate DLB patients with or without disturbances of consciousness with a relative preservation in patients experiencing them[14]. A more recent study has similarly shown discrimination of DLB patients with and without disturbances of consciousness in high-affinity nicotinic receptor binding levels in the thalamus, with patients who are experiencing disturbances in consciousness displaying increased binding in the reticular and ventral anterior thalamic nuclei[26].

GLUTAMATERGIC NEUROTRANSMISSION

There have only been a handful of studies published to date that examine the glutamatergic system in patients with parkinsonian disorders. These studies reported no change in the expression of a glutamate transporter protein in a small number of DLB cases[27], and reduced glutamate receptor immunoreactivity in hippocampus and entorhinal cortex of Lewy body variant of Alzheimer's disease cases[28]. In DLB and Alzheimer's disease cases, a recent study investigated the role of postsynaptic group I metabotropic (mGlu) glutamate receptors, whose function was found to be impaired in the cerebral cortex, due to impairments in receptor signaling and desensitization of group I mGlu receptors[29]. Furthermore, a significant decrease in the expression of the vesicular glutamate (VGLUT) transporter-1 has recently been found in the prefrontal and temporal cortices of Parkinson's disease patients[30], which may have implications in the generation of dementia in Parkinson's disease. Clearly, further studies are required to determine the possible role of glutamatergic neurons in DLB, using a range of pre- and postsynaptic markers now available[3].

DOPAMINERGIC NEUROTRANSMISSION

For DLB and Parkinson's disease, neuronal losses in the substantia nigra from the medial to the lateral region appear to correspond to neuropsychiatric and motor symptoms, respectively. In DLB and idiopathic Parkinson's disease, neuronal loss in this region is correlated with the presence of Lewy pathology. However, in Parkinson's disease, neuronal loss is more asymmetrical than in DLB, leaving the medial region of the substantia nigra less affected in patients with Parkinson's disease[31]. This appears to be reflected in the levels of the dopamine transporter using single photon emission computed tomography (SPECT), which is differentially affected in DLB compared to Alzheimer's disease. While there are some subtle differences between DLB and Parkinson's disease, further work is required for SPECT use in differential diagnosis[32,33]. Differences between DLB and Parkinson's disease in dopaminergic activities are of particular importance due to the differences in the response to levodopa[34] and neuroleptics in DLB and Parkinson's disease patients[35]. Some patients with DLB have a poor response to levodopa treatment and can have a severe reaction to treatment with neuroleptics. This suggests that there may be neuropathologic differences between Parkinson's disease and DLB with respect to dopamine. Piggott and colleagues determined that dopamine D2 receptor levels were significantly reduced (17%) in the caudal putamen in DLB patients compared to controls and patients with Parkinson's disease[36]. In patients with Parkinson's disease, there was an increase in D2 receptors in all coronal sections, especially in the rostral putamen (increase of 71%). This increase in D2 receptors may reflect the unrelenting neurodegeneration of the dopaminergic nigrostriatal pathway seen in Parkinson's disease. In addition, increases in the amount of neuritic pathology in the striatum have been demonstrated in DLB and concomitant Alzheimer's disease/DLB compared to Parkinson's disease[37]. These differences may begin to explain the poor response of some DLB patients to levodopa and do provide a foundation for studying the severe reactions of many DLB patients to neuroleptics. Furthermore, D2 receptors represent an important diagnostic tool to distinguish DLB from Alzheimer's disease[38]. A recent study has investigated the role of thalamic D2 receptors and reported that in both Parkinson's disease and PDD cases, there were significant increases in D2 receptor binding compared to controls, which were not apparent for DLB cases[39].

OTHER NEUROTRANSMITTER SYSTEMS

Changes in serotonergic neurotransmission in Alzheimer's disease include neuron loss and neurofibrillary tangle formation in the raphé nucleus and receptor changes in the neocortex. Recent work indicates a loss of 5HT reuptake sites in the temporal cortex in Alzheimer's disease associated with depression, but with preservation of serotonergic function in the frontal cortex, as indicated by the 5HIAA:5HT ratio[40]. In DLB, Lewy bodies occur in the dorsal raphé nucleus and marked reduction of serotonin levels have been reported in the striatum, neocortex, and frontal cortex. Furthermore, DLB patients with major depression displayed relatively higher binding to the 5HT transporter reuptake sites in the parietal cortex, compared to those without depression. However, while no control data were reported in this study[14], both groups had lower mean values than controls (EK Perry, unpublished observations). In Parkinson's disease, the association between serotonergic dysfunction and depression is clearer, with a number of studies identifying reduced 5HIAA in the cerebrospinal fluid[41,42].

Changes in noradrenergic transmission in Alzheimer's disease and DLB include neuronal loss in the locus ceruleus, although studies have suggested that the surviving noradrenergic neurons may partially compensate for this loss. While hippocampal and cortical levels of noradrenaline are reduced in Alzheimer's disease subjects, these reductions do not appear to correlate well with neuronal loss in the locus ceruleus[43]. A recent *in situ* hybridization study has confirmed decreased expression of α1D and α2c adrenoceptor mRNA in the hippocampus of Alzheimer's disease and DLB cases, although the functional significance of these findings is not yet clear[44].

REFERENCES

1. Duda JE. Pathology and neurotransmitter abnormalities of dementia with Lewy bodies. Dement Geriatr Cogn Disord. 2004;17 Suppl 1:3-14.
2. Francis PT, Palmer AM, Snape M, Wilcock GK. The cholinergic hypothesis of Alzheimer's disease: a review of progress. J Neurol Neurosurg Psychiatry. 1999;66:137-47.
3. Francis PT. Glutamatergic systems in Alzheimer's disease. Int J Geriatr Psychiatry. 2003;18:S15-21.
4. Camicioli R, Moore MM, Kinney A, Corbridge E, Glassberg K, Kaye JA. Parkinson's disease is associated with hippocampal atrophy. Mov Disord. 2003;18:784-90.
5. Laakso MP, Partanen K, Riekkinen P, Lehtovirta M, Helkala EL, Hallikainen M, Hanninen T, Vainio P, Soininen H. Hippocampal volumes in Alzheimer's disease, Parkinson's disease with and without dementia, and in vascular dementia: an MRI study. Neurology. 1996;46:678-81.
6. Burton EJ, McKeith IG, Burn DJ, Williams ED, OBrien JT. Cerebral atrophy in Parkinson's disease with and without dementia: a comparison with Alzheimer's disease, dementia with Lewy bodies and controls. Brain. 2004;127:791-800.
7. Burton EJ, McKeith IG, Burn DJ, O'Brien JT. Brain atrophy rates in Parkinson's disease with and without dementia using serial magnetic resonance imaging. Mov Disord. 2005;20(12):1571-6.

8.	Tsuboi Y, Dickson DW. Dementia with Lewy bodies and Parkinson's disease with dementia: are they different? Parkinsonism Relat Disord. 2005b;11 Suppl 1:S47-51.

9.	Hansen LA, Daniel SE, Wilcock GK, Love S. Frontal cortical synaptophysin in Lewy body diseases: relation to Alzheimer's disease and dementia. J Neurol Neurosurg Psychiatry. 1998;64:653-6.

10.	Perry EK, Kerwin JM, Perry RH, Irving D, Blessed G, Fairbairn AF. Cerebral cholinergic activity is related to the incidence of visual hallucinations in senile dementia of Lewy body type. Dementia. 1990a;1:2-4.

11.	Perry EK, Marshall E, Kerwin J, Smith CJ, Jabeen S, Cheng AV, Perry RH. Evidence of a monoaminergic cholinergic imbalance related to visual hallucinations in Lewy body dementia. J Neurochem. 1990b;55:1454-6.

12.	Tiraboschi P, Hansen LA, Alford M, Merdes A, Masliah E, Thal LJ, Corey-Bloom J. Early and widespread cholinergic losses differentiate dementia with Lewy bodies from Alzheimer disease. Arch Gen Psychiatry. 2002;59:946-51.

13.	Teaktong T, Piggott MA, McKeith IG, Perry RH, Ballard CG, Perry EK. Muscarinic M2 and M4 receptors in anterior cingulate cortex: relation to neuropsychiatric symptoms in dementia with Lewy bodies. Behav Brain Res. 2005;161:299-305.

14.	Ballard C, Piggott M, Johnson M, Cairns N, Perry R, McKeith I, Jaros E, O'Brien J, Holmes C, Perry E. Delusions associated with elevated muscarinic binding in dementia with Lewy bodies. Ann Neurol. 2000;48:868-76.

15.	Hirsch EC, Graybiel AM, Duyckaerts C, Javoy-Agid F. Neuronal loss in the pedunculopontine tegmental nucleus in Parkinson disease and in progressive supranuclear palsy. Proc Natl Acad Sci U S A. 1987;84:5976-80.

16.	Shiozaki K, Iseki E, Uchiyama H, Watanabe Y, Haga T, Kameyama K, Ikeda T, Yamamoto T, Kosaka K. Alterations of muscarinic acetylcholine receptor subtypes in diffuse Lewy body disease: relation to Alzheimer's disease. J Neurol Neurosurg Psychiatry. 1999;67:209-13.

17.	Shiozaki K, Iseki E, Hino H, Kosaka K. Distribution of m1 muscarinic acetylcholine receptors in the hippocampus of patients with Alzheimer's disease and dementia with Lewy bodies-an immunohistochemical study. J Neurol Sci. 2001;193:23-8.

18.	McKeith IG, Grace JB, Walker Z, Byrne EJ, Wilkinson D, Stevens T, Perry EK. Rivastigmine in the treatment of dementia with Lewy bodies: preliminary findings from an open trial. Int J Geriatr Psychiatry. 2000;15:387-92.

19. Perry EK, Morris CM, Court JA, Cheng A, Fairbairn AF, McKeith IG, Irving D, Brown A, Perry RH. Alteration in nicotine binding sites in Parkinson's disease, Lewy body dementia and Alzheimer's: possible index of early neuropathology. Neuroscience. 1995;64:385-95.

20. Martin-Ruiz C, Court J, Lee M, Piggott M, Johnson M, Ballard C, Kalaria R, Perry R, and Perry E. Nicotinic receptors in dementia of Alzheimer, Lewy body and vascular types. Acta Neurol Scand. 2000;Suppl 176:34-41.

21. Reid RT, Sabbagh MN, Corey-Bloom J, Tiraboschi P, Thal LJ. Nicotinic receptor losses in dementia with Lewy bodies: comparisons with Alzheimer's disease. Neurobiol Aging. 2000;21:741-6.

22. Perry E, Martin-Ruiz C, Lee M, Griffiths M, Johnson M, Piggott M, Haroutunian V, Buxbaum JD, Nasland J, Davis K, Gotti C, Clementi F, Tzartos S, Cohen O, Soreq H, Jaros E, Perry R, Ballard C, McKeith I, Court J. Nicotinic receptor subtypes in human brain ageing, Alzheimer and Lewy body diseases. Eur J Pharmacol. 2000;393:215-22.

23. Ray M, Bohr I, McIntosh JM, Ballard C, McKeith I, Chalon S, Guilloteau D, Perry R, Perry E, Court JA, Piggott M. Involvement of alpha6/alpha3 neuronal nicotinic acetylcholine receptors in neuropsychiatric features of Dementia with Lewy bodies: [(125)I]-alpha-conotoxin MII binding in the thalamus and striatum. Neurosci Lett. 2004;372:220-5.

24. Wonnacott S. Presynaptic nicotinic ACh receptors. Trends Neurosci. 1997;20:92-8.

25. Court J, Martin-Ruiz C, Piggott M, Spurden D, Griffiths M, Perry E. Nicotinic receptor abnormalities in Alzheimer's disease. Biol Psychiatry. 2001;49:175-84.

26. Pimlott SL, Piggott M, Ballard C, McKeith I, Perry R, Kometa S, Owens J, Wyper D, Perry E. Thalamic nicotinic receptors implicated in disturbed consciousness in dementia with Lewy bodies. Neurobiol Dis. 2006;21:50-6.

27. Scott HL, Pow DV, Tannenberg AE, Dodd PR. Aberrant expression of the glutamate transporter excitatory amino acid transporter 1 (EAAT1) in Alzheimer's disease. J Neurosci. 2002;22:RC206.

28. Thorns V, Mallory M, Hansen L, Masliah E. Alterations in glutamate receptor 2/3 subunits and amyloid precursor protein expression during the course of Alzheimer's disease and Lewy body variant. Acta Neuropathol (Berl). 1997;94:539-48.

29. Albasanz JL, Dalfo E, Ferrer I, Martin M. Impaired metabotropic glutamate receptor/phospholipase C signaling pathway in the cerebral cortex in Alzheimer's disease and dementia with Lewy bodies correlates with stage of Alzheimer's-disease-related changes. Neurobiol Dis. 2005;20:685-93.

30. Kashani A, Betancur C, Giros B, Hirsch E, Mestikawy SE. Altered expression of vesicular glutamate transporters VGLUT1 and VGLUT2 in Parkinson disease. Neurobiol Aging. 2007;28(4):568-78.

31. Ransmayr G, Seppi K, Donnemiller E, Luginger E, Marksteiner J, Riccabona G, Poewe W, Wenning GK. Striatal dopamine transporter function in dementia with Lewy bodies and Parkinson's disease. Eur J Nucl Med. 2001;28:1523-8.

32. O'Brien JT, Colloby S, Fenwick J, Williams ED, Firbank M, Burn D, Aarsland D, McKeith IG. Dopamine transporter loss visualized with FP-CIT SPECT in the differential diagnosis of dementia with Lewy bodies. Arch Neurol. 2004;61:919-25.

33. Walker Z, Costa DC, Walker RW, Lee L, Livingston G, Jaros E, Perry R, McKeith I, Katona CL. Striatal dopamine transporter in dementia with Lewy bodies and Parkinson disease: a comparison. Neurology. 2004;62:1568-72.

34. McKeith IG, Galasko D, Kosaka K, Perry EK, Dickson DW, Hansen LA, Salmon DP, Lowe J, Mirra SS, Byrne EJ, Lennox G, Quinn NP, Edwardson JA, Ince PG, Bergeron C, Burns A, Miller BL, Lovestone S, Collerton D, Jansen ENH, Ballard C, Devos RAI, Wilcock GK, Jellinger KA, Perry RH. Consensus guidelines for the clinical and pathological diagnosis of dementia with Lewy bodies (DLB) - report of the consortium on DBL international workshop. Neurology. 1996;47:1113-24.

35. Ballard C, Grace J, McKeith I, Holmes C. Neuroleptic sensitivity in dementia with Lewy bodies and Alzheimer's disease. Lancet. 1998;351:1032-3.

36. Piggott MA, Marshall EF, Thomas N, Lloyd S, Court JA, Jaros E, Costa D, Perry RH, Perry EK. Dopaminergic activities in the human striatum: rostrocaudal gradients of uptake sites and of D1 and D2 but not of D3 receptor binding or dopamine. Neuroscience. 1999;90:433-45.

37. Duda JE, Giasson BI, Mabon ME, Lee VM, Trojanowski JQ. Novel antibodies to synuclein show abundant striatal pathology in Lewy body diseases. Ann Neurol. 2002;52:205-10.

38. Walker Z, Costa DC, Janssen AG, Walker RW, Livingstone G, Katona CL. Dementia with Lewy bodies: a study of post-synaptic

dopaminergic receptors with iodine-123 iodobenzamide single-photon emission tomography. Eur J Nucl Med. 1997;24:609-14.

39.   Piggott MA, Ballard CG, Dickinson HO, McKeith IG, Perry RH, Perry EK. Thalamic D2 receptors in dementia with Lewy bodies, Parkinson's disease, and Parkinson's disease dementia. Int J Neuropsychopharmacol. 2007;10(2):231-44.

40.   Chen CP, Alder JT, Bowen DM, Esiri MM, McDonald B, Hope T, Jobst KA, Francis PT. Presynaptic serotonergic markers in community-acquired cases of Alzheimer's disease: correlation with depression and neuroleptic medication. J Neurochem. 1996;66:1592-8.

41.   Kuhn W, Muller T, Gerlach M, Sofic E, Fuchs G, Heye N, Prautsch R, Przuntek H. Depression in Parkinson's disease: biogenic amines in CSF of "de novo" patients. J Neural Transm. 1996;103:1441-5.

42.   Mayeux R, Stern Y, Sano M, Williams JB, Cote LJ. The relationship of serotonin to depression in Parkinson's disease. Mov Disord. 1988;3:237-44.

43.   Hoogendijk WJ, Feenstra MG, Botterblom MH, Gilhuis J, Sommer IE, Kamphorst W, Eikelenboom P, Swaab DF. Increased activity of surviving locus ceruleus neurons in Alzheimer's disease. Ann Neurol. 1999;45:82-91.

44.   Szot P, White SS, Greenup JL, Leverenz JB, Peskind ER, Raskind MA. Compensatory changes in the noradrenergic nervous system in the locus ceruleus and hippocampus of postmortem subjects with Alzheimer's disease and dementia with Lewy bodies. J Neurosci. 2006;26:467-78.

3

Genetic Findings in Parkinson's Disease

Martin Wilhelm Kurz and Dag Aarsland

The Norwegian Centre for Movement Disorders, University Hospital, Stavanger, Norway.

Address correspondence to Dr. M.W. Kurz, Department of Neurology, The Norwegian Centre for Movement Disorders, University Hospital, Stavanger, Postboks 8100, N-4068 Stavanger, Norway.

OUTLINE

Heritability of Parkinson's Disease
Genetic Factors in Parkinson's Disease
    α-Synuclein (PARK1, PARK4)
    Parkin (PARK2)
    Ubiquitin Carboxyl-Terminal Hydrolase L1 (UCH-L1, PARK5)
    PINK1 (PARK6)
    DJ-1 (PARK7)
    LRRK2 (PARK8)
    Further Loci
The Role of Genetics in the Development of Dementia in Parkinson's Disease
References

HERITABILITY OF PARKINSON'S DISEASE

During the last decade, great progress was made in the understanding of the genetic basis and mechanisms of neurological diseases. Particular to the understanding of Parkinson's disease, the recent discovery of genes associated with rare monogenic forms of the disease has provided substantial and novel insight into the molecular disease mechanisms involved. However, in the 1980s, preferred opinion favored environmental toxins as accountable for the disease. This opinion was strengthened by occurrence of Parkinson's disease in people exposed to MPTP (1-methyl 4-phenyl 1,2,3,6-tetrahydro-pyridine), the protective effect of smoking, and the difference between the prevalence of Parkinson's disease in rural and urban areas[1–4]. Early twin studies demonstrated a low rate of concordance in monozygotic and dizygotic twins, further emphasizing an assumed lack of genetic susceptibility[5]. First, in 1999, in an assessment of genetic inheritance in Parkinson's disease by studying the concordance rates of the World War II Veteran Twin Registry, it could be concluded that genetic factors are important when the disease starts at or before the age of 50 years[6]. Further discovery of familial forms of Parkinson's disease and elaboration of the genes involved showed clearly that there was a significant genetic component to the disease[7–9]. Molecular evidence from monogenetic forms of Parkinson's disease promoted substantial insight into the understanding of specific molecular pathways in Parkinson's disease because monogenic and sporadic forms of parkinsonism share many overlapping features[10], implying that common pathogenic mechanisms may underlie disease development.

GENETIC FACTORS IN PARKINSON'S DISEASE

α-Synuclein (PARK1, PARK4)

The first gene coding for familial Parkinson's disease was identified while studying a large kindred from southern Italy (Contursi kindred) with an autosomal-dominant transmission of Parkinson's disease. The gene could be linked to chromosome 4q21-q23[11] and, in 1997, an A53T missense mutation in the *α-synuclein gene* (*SNCA*) was identified as the causative mutation. The mutation consists in the transversion at the nucleotide position 209 from guanine to adenine, leading to the change of alanine to threonine in the mutant protein[12]. Affected individuals had, typically, levodopa-responsive Parkinson's disease with the same clinical features as seen in sporadic disease forms. Some affected individuals developed additionally marked dementia, orthostatic hypotension, bladder incontinence, and myoclonus[13,14]. Since then, two other point mutations in *SNCA* have been elaborated as causative mutations for autosomal-dominant disease transmission. The A30P mutation was found in a German family and involves the substitution of guanine to cytosine at position 88, resulting in the change of alanine to proline[15]. Affected individuals displayed the typical features of levodopa-responsive parkinsonism, except for an early-onset dementia. The E46K mutation was found in a Spanish family[16], and affected carriers usually displayed cognitive decline at an early stage of the disease and showed extensive cortical Lewy body pathology. Recent genetic evidence indicates a direct correlation between *SNCA* dosage and disease progression[17,18], although other studies do not support such a gene dose-behavior relationship hypothesis. There is some indication that variability in the promoter region of *SNCA* can predispose to Parkinson's disease[19].

The α-synuclein protein consists of 140 amino acids and is concentrated in synaptic terminals[20]. The physiological function of α-synuclein is still unknown. Structurally, the amino-terminus contains an amphipathic repeat region that can bind to lipid membranes and associates with presynaptic vesicles[21]. This interaction may play a role in regulating synaptic vesicle size, dopamine storage, and neurotransmission. The A30P mutation causes a loss of liposome binding, leading to a loss of function[22]; the E46K mutation causes an increased liposome binding, leading to assembly into filaments of α-synuclein[23]; and all three mutations lead to an increased self-aggregation and formation of Lewy body–like fibrils[24–27]. One proposed mechanism as to how α-synuclein exerts its neurotoxic effect is through direct impairment of protein degradation over the ubiquitin-proteasome system (UPS)[28]. Other mechanisms have been described as proteasomal inhibition[29] and inhibition of protein degradation over the lysosome/autophagy pathway[30]. Furthermore, overexpression of *α-synuclein* has been linked to mitochondrial dysfunction[31], apoptosis[32], defective cellular trafficking[33], chaperone-mediated autophagy[34], increased sensitivity to oxidative stress[35], and dopamine-mediated toxicity[36].

Parkin (PARK2)

Parkin mutations have been linked first to a rare form of autosomal-recessive, juvenile-onset Parkinson's disease in Japanese families[37,38]. Affected patients display tremor, bradykinesia, rigidity, and have an excellent initial response to levodopa[39,40]. However, some unusual clinical features, such as dystonia at onset, hyperreflexia, and early treatment–related complications, may be present. Furthermore, neuropathological findings are not consistent with idiopathic Parkinson's disease, as Lewy bodies are not found[39,41]. *Parkin* mutations are common in families with early-onset Parkinson's disease and are found in up to 50% of early-onset individuals with a positive family history of Parkinson's disease[42]. In 1998, the gene could be located to chromosome 6q25.2-q27 and a homozygous deletion could be detected[38,43]. Since then, a wide variety of *parkin* mutations have been described, including deletions, multiplications, and missense mutations[44–46]. Although most reported cases show an autosomal-recessive transmission, some cases exist that are not compatible with recessive inheritance, and genetic evidence exists that shows that haploinsufficiency in the *parkin* gene may be a predisposing factor[47,48]. Several studies showed that probands carrying single, defective, *parkin* alleles display reduced 18F-DOPA uptake on positron emission scanning, suggesting a subclinical nigrostriatal dysfunction, thus strengthening the pathogenic relevance of haploinsufficiency[49,50].

Physiologically, *parkin* encodes for a protein consisting of 465 amino acids containing an amino-terminal, ubiquitin-like domain; a central linker region; and a carboxy-terminal RING domain comprising two RING finger motifs separated by an in-between RING domain[51]. Consistent with the RING finger motif, parkin protein acts as an E3 ubiquitin protein ligase[52] in the UPS. Ubiquitination of proteins leads to proteasomal protein degradation. Consequently, parkin mutations should lead to an incorrect ubiquitination and an invalid targeting of the proteasome, leading to protein accumulation. Surprisingly, *parkin* knockout animal models do not show clinical or pathological hallmarks of the disease[53], but proteomic analysis has instead revealed dysfunction in the mitochondrial oxidative phosphorylation in the ventral midbrain[54] and a decrease of mitochondrial respiratory capacity, leading to an increase of oxidative damage[55,56]. Thus, *parkin* may have a neuroprotective effect maintaining mitochondrial integrity. Congruously, overexpression of *parkin* leads to resistance to mitochondrial-dependent apoptosis[57], protection against dopamine-mediated toxicity[58], protection against toxicity induced by proteasomal inhibition[59], and protection against loss of dopaminergic neurons[60].

Ubiquitin Carboxyl-Terminal Hydrolase L1 (UCH-L1, PARK5)

UCH-L1 is a highly abundant, neuron-specific protein involved in the regeneration of monomeric ubiquitin in the UPS[61], functioning as an ubiquitin protein ligase[62] and maintaining ubiquitin homeostasis[63]. A heterozygous mutation (I93M) has been found in an affected German sibling pair[64]. Because the transmitting parent was asymptomatic, the pathogenicity of the mutation is still elusive or an incomplete transmission pattern exists. Additionally, a heterozygous M124L variant was described in an unaffected individual[65]. The common polymorphism S18Y was reported as underrepresented in a European cohort[66] and thus may have a potential protective effect caused by a reduced ligase activity and normal hydrolase activity not leading to α-synuclein accumulation[62]. The protective effect was confirmed in a meta-analysis[67]. However, no other mutations have been identified to date, thus increasing doubts concerning pathogenicity and leading to the suggestion of this being a benign polymorphism[68]. Similarly, mutant mice that lack functional UCH-L1 do not develop a parkinsonian phenotype[64,69], yet a possible pathogenic role of mutations in the *UCH-L1* gene might reduce availability of free ubiquitin monomers, leading to an impaired UPS and protein accumulation[64].

PINK1 (PARK6)

In a large Italian family with familial occurrence of Parkinson's disease, linkage to chromosome 1p36-37 could be accomplished by performing a homozygosity screen[70]. Subsequent mutations in the *PTEN-induced kinase 1 (PINK1)* were identified[71]. Affected individuals display young-onset, but otherwise typical, features of Parkinson's disease. Additional screens of early-onset families revealed various novel mutations. However, *PINK1* mutations remain less common than *parkin* mutations[72,73]. PINK1 is a 581-amino-acid protein containing a mitochondrial targeting motif and a kinase domain homologous to serine/threonine kinases of the calcium/calmodulin family[71]. PINK1 is considered to be a mitochondrial protein with a role in protecting against oxidative stress and apoptosis in *in vitro* models. Accordingly, the G309D mutation is located in the ADP binding site of PINK1 and impairs the protective effect by harming kinase activity[71,74]. However, the kinase activity has yet to be demonstrated, and mitochondrial substrates and interacting proteins have to be identified. PINK1 and parkin seem to cooperate in a common pathway, as overexpression of parkin leads to a complete regression of symptoms caused by PINK1 mutations[75]. Furthermore, genetic evidence exists that haploinsufficiency in the *PINK1* gene may be a predisposing factor, as patients with heterozygous mutations show a 10-year-later disease onset[76], display reduced 18F-DOPA uptake on positron emission scanning[77], and *PINK1* polymorphisms are more frequent among Parkinson's disease patients than in healthy controls[78].

DJ-1 (PARK7)

A homozygosity screen in a family with early-onset Parkinson's disease revealed a linkage to chromosome 1p36[79,80]. Mutations in the gene encoding for the protein DJ-1 were found, including deletions, missense mutations, and splice site alterations[81,82]. Affected individuals have a similar phenotype to those affected with *parkin* mutations, including dystonia at onset and initial good response to levodopa. Some individuals exhibit psychosis. DJ-1 is a homodimeric, 189-amino-acid protein of the DJ-1/ThiJ/PfpI superfamily. The prevalence of *DJ-1* mutations is much lower, accounting for 1–2% of individuals with familial, young-onset Parkinson's disease[83]. DJ-1 is expressed ubiquitously, including the brain, where it is localized to both neurons and glia[84,85]. DJ-1 does not appear in Lewy bodies, but colocalizes with tau-positive inclusions in several neurodegenerative diseases, suggesting a role in distinct neurodegenerative diseases[86,87]. Interestingly, *DJ-1* is depleted in the brains of patients with *parkin* mutations, but enhanced in patients with sporadic Parkinson's disease[88]. The physiological function of DJ-1 is unclear, but it may have a role in protecting against mitochondrial damage in response to oxidative stress[89]. Furthermore, it may protect against endoplasmic reticulum stress and proteasomal inhibition[90]. The L166P mutation that was found in an Italian kindred leads to an unfolding of the carboxy-terminal region and a loss of dimerization, leading to enhanced degradation by the proteasome[85,91]. Additionally, resolution of the dimerization may exhibit direct instability with a consequent abatement of neuroprotective functions[92]. It could be demonstrated that *parkin* associates with mutant DJ-1, supporting its stability[93]. Concordantly, oxidative stress enhances interaction, linking both proteins in a common neuroprotective pathway. It is suggested that DJ-1 may act as a component of the UPS, acting as a chaperone or protease to refold or promote the degradation of misfolded proteins[93].

LRRK2 (PARK8)

A linkage to chromosome 12p11.2-q13.1 in a Japanese family with autosomal-dominant Parkinson's disease has been identified[94]. The findings to date suggest that mutations in the *leucine-rich repeat kinase 2 (LRRK2)* gene are the most common genetic cause of late-onset Parkinson's disease. Until now, frequent mutations have been identified. The most common mutation so far is the G2019S mutation, accounting for 2–6.6% of the autosomal inherited cases with Parkinson's disease, depending on the population investigated[95–98] and 1–2% of the sporadic Parkinson's disease cases[99–101]. It has been suggested that penetrance of *LRRK2* mutations may be age dependent[96,98], explaining the reduced penetrance in some affected families. Furthermore, as *LRRK2* mutations can be seen in asymptomatic individuals and control subjects, an incomplete penetrance is presumed[102]. The R1441G mutation was reported to cause 8% of Parkinson's disease cases in a Basque cohort[99] and the G2019S mutation was not found in any familial Parkinson's disease cases, but only in one out of 337 patients with sporadic Parkinson's disease[103]. However, this mutation was present in 41% of probands with autosomal-dominant Parkinson's disease, mostly from France and North Africa[104], indicating different frequencies of specific *LRRK2* mutations in different populations. Affected individuals exhibit a clinical phenotype compatible with idiopathic Parkinson's disease, but show a wide variety of neuropathological patterns, ranging from pure degeneration without Lewy bodies to degeneration with brainstem Lewy bodies, widespread Lewy bodies with a distribution similar the distribution in dementia with Lewy bodies (DLB), and neurofibrillary tau-positive tangles[94,105,106]. However, the prevalence of cognitive dysfunction and dementia among *LRRK2* mutation carriers is surprisingly low, although the G2019S mutation is located on chromosome 12q12, a genetic locus implicated in late-onset Alzheimer's disease[107].

At present, it still has to be determined how mutations in the *LRRK2* gene cause Parkinson's disease. The *LRRK2* gene contains 51 exons and encodes a protein consisting of 2527 amino acids called dardarin[99]. The protein comprises various, highly conserved domains with probable functional attributes and, so far, it is unclear which domains play a relevant role in neurodegeneration.

Further Loci

PARK3 is a genetic locus for autosomal-dominant Parkinson's disease linked to chromosome 2p13, described in two American families descending from southern Denmark/Northern Germany[108,109]. Penetrance of the mutation is reduced and gene mutations may be widely distributed in the population. Age at onset is similar to sporadic Parkinson's disease.

PARK10 and *PARK11* have been defined in large population samples and linked to chromosome 1p32 *(PARK10)*[110] and 2q36-q37 *(PARK11)*[111]. These loci represent susceptibility loci, which may be important in the pathogenesis of sporadic Parkinson's disease.

NURR1 (NR4A2) is a developmental gene that is important in development and maintenance of midbrain dopaminergic neurons. Two mutations have been found in exon 1 and linkage could be done to chromosome 2q22-q23[112–114]. At present, linkage has not been described in a single large family and findings could not be replicated. Pathogenic relevance has to be determined.

Synphilin-1 (SNCAIP) is a substrate of the gene product of *parkin* and has been shown to interact directly with α-synuclein[115]. It is found in Lewy bodies along with parkin and α-synuclein. Linkage could be done to chromosome 5q23.1-q23.3[116]. A direct role for *synphilin-1* is suggested by identification of the R621C mutation in two, apparently sporadic, Parkinson's disease patients of German origin. Both patients reported no family history of Parkinson's disease, but genotyping suggested a common ancestor. Functional studies showed that mutant synphilin can form cytoplasmic inclusions. Furthermore, transfected cells carrying the R621C mutation are more susceptible to apoptosis than normal control cells.

Candidate genes identified on the basis of their involvement in the dopamine pathway have been proposed as susceptibility genes, including *MAO B, dopamine D2 receptor, CYP2D6, CYP1A1, N-acetyltransferase 2, DAT1,* and *glutathione S-transferase M1*[117–119]. Until now, the few studies with significant associations between candidate genes and Parkinson's disease have failed to replicate in other samples. Thus, the pathological relevance of those candidate genes has to be examined further.

Mitochondrial dysfunction has been implicated in the pathogenesis of Parkinson's disease for a long time. A majority of mitochondrial DNA is dedicated to the reduced nicotin-amide adenine dinucleotide complex I enzyme; thus, mitochondrial DNA variation might contribute to Parkinson's disease expression. Ten, single, nucleotide polymorphisms defining European mitochondrial DNA haplogroups were genotyped in Caucasian Parkinson's disease patients and controls. Haplotype J or K was significantly lower associated with Parkinson's disease than hapolotype H, suggesting that variation in complex I proteins may be a risk factor for Parkinson's disease[120].

Until now, genetic Parkinson's disease cases explain no more than 5–10% of the overall Parkinson's disease population. Thus, the relationship between pathogenic principles of familial Parkinson's disease and the common sporadic form remains a key problem in the interpretation of devised results. However, both familial and sporadic forms of the disease overlap in their clinical syndrome and their characteristic pathology. Hence, the understanding of the molecular basis of genetically caused Parkinson's disease may contribute significantly to the understanding of the molecular biology of both familial and sporadic Parkinson's disease cases with important therapeutic potential for the patients.

THE ROLE OF GENETICS IN DEVELOPMENT OF DEMENTIA IN PARKINSON'S DISEASE

Parkinson's disease has traditionally been assumed to be mainly a motor disorder. However, in the past few years, dementia in Parkinson's disease has been recognized increasingly and a cumulative frequency of dementia in Parkinson's disease as high as 78% has been reported[121]. The clinical relevance of this issue is emphasized by the observation that the increased mortality risk in Parkinson's disease is ascribed largely to the increased risk of becoming demented[122]. Over the last decade, enormous advances have been achieved in the understanding of the molecular basis of Alzheimer's disease, the most common cause of dementia. Several genes have been identified, such as presenilin 1 and 2, apolipoprotein e (ApoE), and amyloid precursor protein involved in the development of Alzheimer's disease. In parallel, progress in the genetics of Parkinson's disease has enhanced our understanding of basic disease mechanisms in Parkinson's disease, highlighting the role of α-synuclein (see above).

Two main entities that classify dementia in Parkinson's disease are differentiated according to current diagnostic criteria. Parkinson's disease dementia (PDD) is diagnosed if cognitive decline appears more than 1 year subsequent to motor symptoms of Parkinson's disease, and DLB is diagnosed if dementia precedes motor symptoms or occurs within 1 year after motor onset of Parkinson's disease[123]. DLB is seen as a distinct clinical entity characterized clinically by parkinsonism; visual hallucinations; and fluctuating, cognitive impairment; in addition to a dementia syndrome dominated by attentional, executive, and visuospatial deficits and with relatively preserved memory early in course.

In a systematic review of the available literature in respect of familial occurrence and genetics of dementia plus parkinsonism, in order to explore the genetic evidence of PDD and DLB, we found substantial coincidental familial occurrence of dementia and parkinsonism in 24 families[124]. In 12 families, the presentation of dementia and parkinsonism fulfilled current criteria for DLB and PDD, implying that the same mutation in different members of the same family caused different clinical entities. This demonstrates a substantial overlap between the entities in at least a proportion of the cases, suggesting a shared underlying pathophysiology of PDD and DLB. Furthermore, it implies that the arbitrary distinction between PDD and DLB according to the relative timing of parkinsonism and dementia does not reflect the molecular biology of the disease process. As this overlap is clearly evident in familial cases of PDD or DLB, it is likely that the same will be true in sporadic presentations. Interestingly, patients with familial cooccurrence of dementia and parkinsonism displayed either mutations in the synuclein gene or showed positive correlations with the ApoE ε3/4 and ε4/4 allele.

α-Synuclein is the main component of the Lewy bodies, underlining the pathogenic relevance of α-synuclein in familial and sporadic forms of the disease. Accumulation of Lewy bodies shows genetic determinants[25,125], thus development of dementia in Parkinson's disease should be conclusively influenced by them as well. Furthermore, because a direct relationship between extension of Lewy bodies and degree of dementia in Parkinson's disease could be shown[126], the hypothesis that α-synuclein accumulation is also a key factor in development of dementia in Parkinson's disease is additionally strengthened. Since *SNCA* dosage has been found to be correlated to disease progression directly[17,18], it is reasonable to suggest that degree of genetic alteration is determining clinical severity, i.e., time to development of dementia. However, despite the pathogenic relevance of α-synuclein, mutations in the *SNCA* remain a rare cause for familial forms of Parkinson's disease[127].

ApoE is a polymorphic protein that is involved in lipid transport, immunoregulation, and modulation of cell growth[128]. It is abundant in the brain and coded by the *ApoE* gene located on chromosome 19q13.2. The gene is polymorphic, with three major alleles (ε2, ε3, and ε4) yielding six possible genotypes and translating into three major isoforms of the protein: ApoE2, ApoE3, and ApoE4. These isoforms differ from each other only by single amino acid substitutions at position 112 and 158 of the protein, but have far-reaching physiological implications. The ApoE ε3 is the most common allele. About 95% of the normal Caucasian population carry at least one ε3 allele[129]. The ε2 allele is associated with hyperlipoproteinemia[130] and is considered protective in Alzheimer's disease[128]. Congruously, it has been demonstrated to facilitate neurite outgrowth[128] and to inhibit apoptosis[131]. The ε4 allele is associated with an increased risk of developing Alzheimer's disease and a lower age at disease onset[132–134]. Evidence for the role of ApoE in Parkinson's disease has been inconclusive. Contradicting studies have shown associations of Parkinson's disease with the ε2 allele[135,136] and of the ε4 allele with Parkinson's disease[137], PDD[122,138–140], and hallucinations or psychosis in Parkinson's disease[141]. Other studies failed to show significant associations[142,143]. Furthermore, an inverse association between the ε3 allele and PDD has been observed[140]. Interestingly, analyses including larger sample sizes elaborated a significant association of the ε4 allele with early age of onset in Parkinson's disease[138,144,145]. However, other studies failed to show this association[139,146] and competing effects, such as sample size limitations, differing ethnicities, and publication bias (unpublished negative studies), must be taken into consideration. Yet, as larger studies and meta-analyses can show a positive association between ApoE ε4 allele and dementia in Parkinson's disease, influence of the ε4 allele has a profound probability. However, the mechanisms by which the ApoE allele may influence the development of Lewy bodies and dementia in Alzheimer's disease and Parkinson's disease remain elusive. Pathologically, both diseases comprise the accumulation of insoluble protein deposits and it is suggested that pathologic cascades that lead to protein accumulation may operate synergistically in some cases[147]. As further significant associations in other neuro-degenerative diseases (such as amyotrophic lateral sclerosis[148] or macular degeneration[149]) exist, occurrence of common principles in different neurodegenerative disorders is further strengthened.

A genetic contribution to PDD is further strengthened by the fact that familial occurrence of Parkinson's disease in first- and second-degree relatives was associated with occurrence of dementia in Parkinson's disease. This association showed a relation to strength of family association, indicating a possible gene dose-dependent effect[150].

Detection of mutations in *LRRK2* gene[99,100] has complicated interpretation. The findings to date suggest that mutations in the LRRK2 gene are the most common genetic cause for late-onset Parkinson's disease (see above). Affected individuals display clinical findings typical for sporadic Parkinson's disease without major development of dementia[103]. The pathomorphologic picture, however, is remarkably varying, ranging from pure degeneration without Lewy bodies to degeneration with brainstem Lewy bodies, widespread Lewy bodies fitting to the pattern seen in DLB, and neurofibrillary tau-positive tangles[105,151]. The mechanisms by which mutations in the *LRRK2* gene cause Parkinson's disease and the reason why neuropathologic patterns fitting those of DLB are not accompanied by dementia still have to be determined. Consequently, other influences like neurochemical effects as the cholinergic deficit have to influence as well, leading to the typical clinical picture with early dementia and development of neuropsychiatric deficits.

The evidence from genetic studies of Parkinson's disease is pointing to a substantial genetic contribution in the pathogenesis of Parkinson's disease, as linkage analyses and positional cloning provided an increasing number of genes involved in the pathogenesis (see above). Furthermore, it is increasingly apparent that there exists a genetic contribution to disease progression and coincidental development of dementia and psychosis in Parkinson's disease. Clearly, in the future, larger and statistically more powerful studies are needed to validate the mode of genetic participation and to explore the underlying processes at the molecular level involved.

The aim of the study of genetics should be to define a sufficient therapy aimed at the pathogenesis of the disease. Thus, the emerging challenge will be the transfer of molecular insight to clinical practice.

REFERENCES

1. Langston JW, Ballard P, Tetrud JW, Irwin I. Chronic parkinsonism in humans due to a product of meperidine-analog synthesis. Science. 1983;219:979-80.
2. Langston JW, Irwin I. MPTP: current concepts and controversies. Clin Neuropharmacol. 1986;9:485-507.
3. Tanner CM. The role of environmental toxins in the etiology of Parkinson's disease. Trends Neurosci. 1989;12:49-54.
4. Alves G, Kurz M, Lie SA, Larsen JP. Cigarette smoking in Parkinson's disease: influence on disease progression. Mov Disord. 2004;19:1087-92.
5. Ward CD, Duvoisin RC, Ince SE, Nutt JD, Eldridge R, Calne DB. Parkinson's disease in 65 pairs of twins and in a set of quadruplets. Neurology. 1983;33:815-24.
6. Tanner CM, Ottman R, Goldman SM, Ellenberg J, Chan P, Mayeux R, Langston JW. Parkinson disease in twins: an etiologic study. JAMA. 1999;281:341-6.
7. Marder K, Tang MX, Mejia H, Alfaro B, Cote L, Louis E, Groves J, Mayeux R. Risk of Parkinson's disease among first-degree relatives: a community-based study. Neurology. 1996;47:155-60.
8. Sveinbjornsdottir S, Hicks AA, Jonsson T, Petursson H, Gugmundsson G, Frigge ML, Kong A, Gulcher JR, Stefansson K.

Familial aggregation of Parkinson's disease in Iceland. N Engl J Med. 2000;343:1765-70.

9. Kurz M, Alves G, Aarsland D, Larsen JP. Familial Parkinson's disease: a community-based study. Eur J Neurol. 2003;10:159-63.

10. Hardy J. Impact of genetic analysis on Parkinson's disease research. Mov Disord. 2003;18 Suppl 6:S96-8.

11. Polymeropoulos MH, Higgins JJ, Golbe LI, Johnson WG, Ide SE, Di Iorio G, Sanges G, Stenroos ES, Pho LT, Schaffer AA, Lazzarini AM, Nussbaum RL, Duvoisin RC. Mapping of a gene for Parkinson's disease to chromosome 4q21-q23. Science. 1996;274:1197-9.

12. Polymeropoulos MH, Lavedan C, Leroy E, Ide SE, Dehejia A, Dutra A, Pike B, Root H, Rubenstein J, Boyer R, Stenroos ES, Chandrasekharappa S, Athanassiadou A, Papapetropoulos T, Johnson WG, Lazzarini AM, Duvoisin RC, Di Iorio G, Golbe LI, Nussbaum RL. Mutation in the alpha-synuclein gene identified in families with Parkinson's disease. Science. 1997;276:2045-7.

13. Golbe LI, Di Iorio G, Sanges G, Lazzarini AM, La Sala S, Bonavita V, Duvoisin RC. Clinical genetic analysis of Parkinson's disease in the Contursi kindred. Ann Neurol. 1996;40:767-75.

14. Spira PJ, Sharpe DM, Halliday G, Cavanagh J, Nicholson GA. Clinical and pathological features of a Parkinsonian syndrome in a family with an Ala53Thr alpha-synuclein mutation. Ann Neurol. 2001;49:313-9.

15. Kruger R, Kuhn W, Muller T, Woitalla D, Graeber M, Kosel S, Przuntek H, Epplen JT, Schols L, Riess O. Ala30Pro mutation in the gene encoding alpha-synuclein in Parkinson's disease. Nat Genet. 1998;18:106-8.

16. Zarranz JJ, Alegre J, Gomez-Esteban JC, Lezcano E, Ros R, Ampuero I, Vidal L, Hoenicka J, Rodriguez O, Atares B, Llorens V, Gomez Tortosa E, del Ser T, Munoz DG, de Yebenes JG. The new mutation, E46K, of alpha-synuclein causes Parkinson and Lewy body dementia. Ann Neurol. 2004;55:164-73.

17. Singleton AB, Farrer M, Johnson J, Singleton A, Hague S, Kachergus J, Hulihan M, Peuralinna T, Dutra A, Nussbaum R, Lincoln S, Crawley A, Hanson M, Maraganore D, Adler C, Cookson MR, Muenter M, Baptista M, Miller D, Blancato J, Hardy J, Gwinn-Hardy K. alpha-Synuclein locus triplication causes Parkinson's disease. Science. 2003;302:841.

18. Chartier-Harlin MC, Kachergus J, Roumier C, Mouroux V, Douay X, Lincoln S, Levecque C, Larvor L, Andrieux J, Hulihan M, Waucquier N, Defebvre L, Amouyel P, Farrer M, Destee A. Alpha-synuclein

locus duplication as a cause of familial Parkinson's disease. Lancet. 2004;364:1167-9.

19. Pals P, Lincoln S, Manning J, Heckman M, Skipper L, Hulihan M, Van den Broeck M, De Pooter T, Cras P, Crook J, Van Broeckhoven C, Farrer MJ. alpha-Synuclein promoter confers susceptibility to Parkinson's disease. Ann Neurol. 2004;56:591-5.

20. Goedert M. Parkinson's disease and other alpha-synucleinopathies. Clin Chem Lab Med. 2001;39:308-12.

21. Outeiro TF, Lindquist S. Yeast cells provide insight into alpha-synuclein biology and pathobiology. Science. 2003;302:1772-5.

22. Bussell R Jr, Eliezer D. Effects of Parkinson's disease-linked mutations on the structure of lipid-associated alpha-synuclein. Biochemistry. 2004;43:4810-8.

23. Choi W, Zibaee S, Jakes R, Serpell LC, Davletov B, Crowther RA, Goedert M. Mutation E46K increases phospholipid binding and assembly into filaments of human alpha-synuclein. FEBS Lett. 2004;576:363-8.

24. Li J, Uversky VN, Fink AL. Conformational behavior of human alpha-synuclein is modulated by familial Parkinson's disease point mutations A30P and A53T. Neurotoxicology. 2002;23:553-67.

25. Kotzbauer PT, Giasson BI, Kravitz AV, Golbe LI, Mark MH, Trojanowski JQ, Lee VM. Fibrillization of alpha-synuclein and tau in familial Parkinson's disease caused by the A53T alpha-synuclein mutation. Exp Neurol. 2004;187:279-88.

26. Greenbaum EA, Graves CL, Mishizen-Eberz AJ, Lupoli MA, Lynch DR, Englander SW, Axelsen PH, Giasson BI. The E46K mutation in alpha-synuclein increases amyloid fibril formation. J Biol Chem. 2005;280:7800-7.

27. Pandey N, Schmidt RE, Galvin JE. The alpha-synuclein mutation E46K promotes aggregation in cultured cells. Exp Neurol. 2006;197:515-20.

28. Eriksen JL, Wszolek Z, Petrucelli L. Molecular pathogenesis of Parkinson disease. Arch Neurol. 2005;62:353-7.

29. McNaught KS, Perl DP, Brownell AL, Olanow CW. Systemic exposure to proteasome inhibitors causes a progressive model of Parkinson's disease. Ann Neurol. 2004;56:149-62.

30. Webb JL, Ravikumar B, Atkins J, Skepper JN, Rubinsztein DC. Alpha-Synuclein is degraded by both autophagy and the proteasome. J Biol Chem. 2003;278:25009-13.

31. Hsu LJ, Sagara Y, Arroyo A, Rockenstein E, Sisk A, Mallory M, Wong J, Takenouchi T, Hashimoto M, Masliah E. alpha-synuclein promotes

mitochondrial deficit and oxidative stress. Am J Pathol. 2000;157:401-10.

32. Lee FJ, Liu F, Pristupa ZB, Niznik HB. Direct binding and functional coupling of alpha-synuclein to the dopamine transporters accelerate dopamine-induced apoptosis. FASEB J. 2001;15:916-26.

33. Gosavi N, Lee HJ, Lee JS, Patel S, Lee SJ. Golgi fragmentation occurs in the cells with prefibrillar alpha-synuclein aggregates and precedes the formation of fibrillar inclusion. J Biol Chem. 2002;277:48984-92.

34. Cuervo AM, Stefanis L, Fredenburg R, Lansbury PT, Sulzer D. Impaired degradation of mutant alpha-synuclein by chaperone-mediated autophagy. Science. 2004;305:1292-5.

35. Ko L, Mehta ND, Farrer M, Easson C, Hussey J, Yen S, Hardy J, Yen SH. Sensitization of neuronal cells to oxidative stress with mutated human alpha-synuclein. J Neurochem. 2000;75:2546-54.

36. Tabrizi SJ, Orth M, Wilkinson JM, Taanman JW, Warner TT, Cooper JM, Schapira AH. Expression of mutant alpha-synuclein causes increased susceptibility to dopamine toxicity. Hum Mol Genet. 2000;9:2683-9.

37. Matsumine H, Saito M, Shimoda-Matsubayashi S, Tanaka H, Ishikawa A, Nakagawa-Hattori Y, Yokochi M, Kobayashi T, Igarashi S, Takano H, Sanpei K, Koike R, Mori H, Kondo T, Mizutani Y, Schaffer AA, Yamamura Y, Nakamura S, Kuzuhara S, Tsuji S, Mizuno Y. Localization of a gene for an autosomal recessive form of juvenile Parkinsonism to chromosome 6q25.2-27. Am J Hum Genet. 1997;60:588-96.

38. Kitada T, Asakawa S, Hattori N, Matsumine H, Yamamura Y, Minoshima S, Yokochi M, Mizuno Y, Shimizu N. Mutations in the parkin gene cause autosomal recessive juvenile parkinsonism. Nature. 1998;392:605-8.

39. Takahashi H, Ohama E, Suzuki S, Horikawa Y, Ishikawa A, Morita T, Tsuji S, Ikuta F. Familial juvenile parkinsonism: clinical and pathologic study in a family. Neurology. 1994;44:437-41.

40. Ishikawa A, Tsuji S. Clinical analysis of 17 patients in 12 Japanese families with autosomal-recessive type juvenile parkinsonism. Neurology. 1996;47:160-6.

41. Mori H, Kondo T, Yokochi M, Matsumine H, Nakagawa-Hattori Y, Miyake T, Suda K, Mizuno Y. Pathologic and biochemical studies of juvenile parkinsonism linked to chromosome 6q. Neurology. 1998;51:890-2.

42. Lucking CB, Durr A, Bonifati V, Vaughan J, De Michele G, Gasser T, Harhangi BS, Meco G, Denefle P, Wood NW, Agid Y, Brice A.

Association between early-onset Parkinson's disease and mutations in the parkin gene. N Engl J Med. 2000;342:1560-7.

43. Matsumine H, Yamamura Y, Hattori N, Kobayashi T, Kitada T, Yoritaka A, Mizuno Y. A microdeletion of D6S305 in a family of autosomal recessive juvenile parkinsonism (PARK2). Genomics. 1998;49:143-6.

44. Farrer MJ. Genetics of Parkinson disease: paradigm shifts and future prospects. Nat Rev Genet. 2006;7:306-18.

45. West AB, Maidment NT. Genetics of parkin-linked disease. Hum Genet. 2004;114:327-36.

46. Mata IF, Lockhart PJ, Farrer MJ. Parkin genetics: one model for Parkinson's disease. Hum Mol Genet. 2004;13(Spec No 1):R127-33.

47. Foroud T, Uniacke SK, Liu L, Pankratz N, Rudolph A, Halter C, Shults C, Marder K, Conneally PM, Nichols WC. Heterozygosity for a mutation in the parkin gene leads to later onset Parkinson disease. Neurology. 2003;60:796-801.

48. Oliveira SA, Scott WK, Martin ER, Nance MA, Watts RL, Hubble JP, Koller WC, Pahwa R, Stern MB, Hiner BC, Ondo WG, Allen FH Jr, Scott BL, Goetz CG, Small GW, Mastaglia F, Stajich JM, Zhang F, Booze MW, Winn MP, Middleton LT, Haines JL, Pericak-Vance MA, Vance JM. Parkin mutations and susceptibility alleles in late-onset Parkinson's disease. Ann Neurol. 2003;53:624-9.

49. Khan NL, Horta W, Eunson L, Graham E, Johnson JO, Chang S, Davis M, Singleton A, Wood NW, Lees AJ. Parkin disease in a Brazilian kindred: manifesting heterozygotes and clinical follow-up over 10 years. Mov Disord. 2005;20:479-84.

50. Khan NL, Scherfler C, Graham E, Bhatia KP, Quinn N, Lees AJ, Brooks DJ, Wood NW, Piccini P. Dopaminergic dysfunction in unrelated, asymptomatic carriers of a single parkin mutation. Neurology. 2005;64:134-6.

51. Moore DJ, West AB, Dawson VL, Dawson TM. Molecular pathophysiology of Parkinson's disease. Annu Rev Neurosci. 2005;28:57-87.

52. Shimura H, Hattori N, Kubo S, Mizuno Y, Asakawa S, Minoshima S, Shimizu N, Iwai K, Chiba T, Tanaka K, Suzuki T. Familial Parkinson disease gene product, parkin, is a ubiquitin-protein ligase. Nat Genet. 2000;25:302-5.

53. Goldberg MS, Fleming SM, Palacino JJ, Cepeda C, Lam HA, Bhatnagar A, Meloni EG, Wu N, Ackerson LC, Klapstein GJ, Gajendiran M, Roth BL, Chesselet MF, Maidment NT, Levine MS,

Shen J. Parkin-deficient mice exhibit nigrostriatal deficits but not loss of dopaminergic neurons. J Biol Chem. 2003;278:43628-35.

54. Palacino JJ, Sagi D, Goldberg MS, Krauss S, Motz C, Wacker M, Klose J, Shen J. Mitochondrial dysfunction and oxidative damage in parkin-deficient mice. J Biol Chem. 2004;279:18614-22.

55. Greene JC, Whitworth AJ, Kuo I, Andrews LA, Feany MB, Pallanck LJ. Mitochondrial pathology and apoptotic muscle degeneration in Drosophila parkin mutants. Proc Natl Acad Sci U S A. 2003;100:4078-83.

56. Pesah Y, Pham T, Burgess H, Middlebrooks B, Verstreken P, Zhou Y, Harding M, Bellen H, Mardon G. Drosophila parkin mutants have decreased mass and cell size and increased sensitivity to oxygen radical stress. Development. 2004;131:2183-94.

57. Darios F, Corti O, Lucking CB, Hampe C, Muriel MP, Abbas N, Gu WJ, Hirsch EC, Rooney T, Ruberg M, Brice A. Parkin prevents mitochondrial swelling and cytochrome c release in mitochondria-dependent cell death. Hum Mol Genet. 2003;12:517-26.

58. Jiang H, Ren Y, Zhao J, Feng J. Parkin protects human dopaminergic neuroblastoma cells against dopamine-induced apoptosis. Hum Mol Genet. 2004;13:1745-54.

59. Petrucelli L, O'Farrell C, Lockhart PJ, Baptista M, Kehoe K, Vink L, Choi P, Wolozin B, Farrer M, Hardy J, Cookson MR. Parkin protects against the toxicity associated with mutant alpha-synuclein: proteasome dysfunction selectively affects catecholaminergic neurons. Neuron. 2002;36:1007-19.

60. Yang Y, Nishimura I, Imai Y, Takahashi R, Lu B. Parkin suppresses dopaminergic neuron-selective neurotoxicity induced by Pael-R in Drosophila. Neuron. 2003;37:911-24.

61. Wilkinson KD, Lee KM, Deshpande S, Duerksen-Hughes P, Boss JM, Pohl J. The neuron-specific protein PGP 9.5 is a ubiquitin carboxyl-terminal hydrolase. Science. 1989;246:670-3.

62. Liu Y, Fallon L, Lashuel HA, Liu Z, Lansbury PT Jr. The UCH-L1 gene encodes two opposing enzymatic activities that affect alpha-synuclein degradation and Parkinson's disease susceptibility. Cell. 2002;111:209-18.

63. Osaka H, Wang YL, Takada K, Takizawa S, Setsuie R, Li H, Sato Y, Nishikawa K, Sun YJ, Sakurai M, Harada T, Hara Y, Kimura I, Chiba S, Namikawa K, Kiyama H, Noda M, Aoki S, Wada K. Ubiquitin carboxy-terminal hydrolase L1 binds to and stabilizes monoubiquitin in neuron. Hum Mol Genet. 2003;12:1945-58.

64. Leroy E, Boyer R, Auburger G, Leube B, Ulm G, Mezey E, Harta G, Brownstein MJ, Jonnalagada S, Chernova T, Dehejia A, Lavedan C, Gasser T, Steinbach PJ, Wilkinson KD, Polymeropoulos MH. The ubiquitin pathway in Parkinson's disease. Nature. 1998;395:451-2.

65. Farrer M, Destee T, Becquet E, Wavrant-De Vrieze F, Mouroux V, Richard F, Defebvre L, Lincoln S, Hardy J, Amouyel P, Chartier-Harlin MC. Linkage exclusion in French families with probable Parkinson' s disease. Mov Disord. 2000;15:1075-83.

66. Maraganore DM, Farrer MJ, Hardy JA, Lincoln SJ, McDonnell SK, Rocca WA. Case-control study of the ubiquitin carboxy-terminal hydrolase L1 gene in Parkinson's disease. Neurology. 1999;53:1858-60.

67. Maraganore DM, Lesnick TG, Elbaz A, Chartier-Harlin MC, Gasser T, Kruger R, Hattori N, Mellick GD, Quattrone A, Satoh J, Toda T, Wang J, Ioannidis JP, de Andrade M, Rocca WA. UCHL1 is a Parkinson's disease susceptibility gene. Ann Neurol. 2004;55:512-21.

68. Lincoln S, Vaughan J, Wood N, Baker M, Adamson J, Gwinn-Hardy K, Lynch T, Hardy J, Farrer M. Low frequency of pathogenic mutations in the ubiquitin carboxy-terminal hydrolase gene in familial Parkinson's disease. Neuroreport. 1999;10:427-9.

69. Saigoh K, Wang YL, Suh JG, Yamanishi T, Sakai Y, Kiyosawa H, Harada T, Ichihara N, Wakana S, Kikuchi T, Wada K. Intragenic deletion in the gene encoding ubiquitin carboxy-terminal hydrolase in gad mice. Nat Genet. 1999;23:47-51.

70. Valente EM, Bentivoglio AR, Dixon PH, Ferraris A, Ialongo T, Frontali M, Albanese A, Wood NW. Localization of a novel locus for autosomal recessive early-onset parkinsonism, PARK6, on human chromosome 1p35-p36. Am J Hum Genet. 2001;68:895-900.

71. Valente EM, Abou-Sleiman PM, Caputo V, Muqit MM, Harvey K, Gispert S, Ali Z, Del Turco D, Bentivoglio AR, Healy DG, Albanese A, Nussbaum R, Gonzalez-Maldonado R, Deller T, Salvi S, Cortelli P, Gilks WP, Latchman DS, Harvey RJ, Dallapiccola B, Auburger G, Wood NW. Hereditary early-onset Parkinson's disease caused by mutations in PINK1. Science. 2004;304:1158-60.

72. Valente EM, Salvi S, Ialongo T, Marongiu R, Elia AE, Caputo V, Romito L, Albanese A, Dallapiccola B, Bentivoglio AR. PINK1 mutations are associated with sporadic early-onset parkinsonism. Ann Neurol. 2004;56:336-41.

73. Hatano Y, Sato K, Elibol B, Yoshino H, Yamamura Y, Bonifati V, Shinotoh H, Asahina M, Kobayashi S, Ng AR, Rosales RL, Hassin-Baer S, Shinar Y, Lu CS, Chang HC, Wu-Chou YH, Atac FB, Kobayashi T, Toda T, Mizuno Y, Hattori N. PARK6-linked autosomal

recessive early-onset parkinsonism in Asian populations. Neurology. 2004;63:1482-5.

74. Bossy-Wetzel E, Schwarzenbacher R, Lipton SA. Molecular pathways to neurodegeneration. Nat Med. 2004;10 Suppl:S2-9.

75. Clark IE, Dodson MW, Jiang C, Cao JH, Huh JR, Seol JH, Yoo SJ, Hay BA, Guo M. Drosophila pink1 is required for mitochondrial function and interacts genetically with parkin. Nature. 2006;441:1162-6.

76. Bonifati V, Rohe CF, Breedveld GJ, Fabrizio E, De Mari M, Tassorelli C, Tavella A, Marconi R, Nicholl DJ, Chien HF, Fincati E, Abbruzzese G, Marini P, De Gaetano A, Horstink MW, Maat-Kievit JA, Sampaio C, Antonini A, Stocchi F, Montagna P, Toni V, Guidi M, Dalla Libera A, Tinazzi M, De Pandis F, Fabbrini G, Goldwurm S, de Klein A, Barbosa E, Lopiano L, Martignoni E, Lamberti P, Vanacore N, Meco G, Oostra BA. Early-onset parkinsonism associated with PINK1 mutations: frequency, genotypes, and phenotypes. Neurology. 2005;65:87-95.

77. Khan NL, Valente EM, Bentivoglio AR, Wood NW, Albanese A, Brooks DJ, Piccini P. Clinical and subclinical dopaminergic dysfunction in PARK6-linked parkinsonism: an 18F-dopa PET study. Ann Neurol. 2002;52:849-53.

78. Abou-Sleiman PM, Muqit MM, McDonald NQ, Yang YX, Gandhi S, Healy DG, Harvey K, Harvey RJ, Deas E, Bhatia K, Quinn N, Lees A, Latchman DS, Wood NW. A heterozygous effect for PINK1 mutations in Parkinson's disease? Ann Neurol. 2006;60:414-9.

79. van Duijn CM, Dekker MC, Bonifati V, Galjaard RJ, Houwing-Duistermaat JJ, Snijders PJ, Testers L, Breedveld GJ, Horstink M, Sandkuijl LA, van Swieten JC, Oostra BA, Heutink P. Park7, a novel locus for autosomal recessive early-onset parkinsonism, on chromosome 1p36. Am J Hum Genet. 2001;69:629-34.

80. Bonifati V, Dekker MC, Vanacore N, Fabbrini G, Squitieri F, Marconi R, Antonini A, Brustenghi P, Dalla Libera A, De Mari M, Stocchi F, Montagna P, Gallai V, Rizzu P, van Swieten JC, Oostra B, van Duijn CM, Meco G, Heutink P. Autosomal recessive early onset parkinsonism is linked to three loci: PARK2, PARK6, and PARK7. Neurol Sci. 2002;23 Suppl 2:S59-60.

81. Bonifati V, Rizzu P, Squitieri F, Krieger E, Vanacore N, van Swieten JC, Brice A, van Duijn CM, Oostra B, Meco G, Heutink P. DJ-1(PARK7), a novel gene for autosomal recessive, early onset parkinsonism. Neurol Sci. 2003;24:159-60.

82. Bonifati V, Oostra BA, Heutink P. Linking DJ-1 to neurodegeneration offers novel insights for understanding the pathogenesis of Parkinson's disease. J Mol Med. 2004;82:163-74.

83. Hedrich K, Djarmati A, Schafer N, Hering R, Wellenbrock C, Weiss PH, Hilker R, Vieregge P, Ozelius LJ, Heutink P, Bonifati V, Schwinger E, Lang AE, Noth J, Bressman SB, Pramstaller PP, Riess O, Klein C. DJ-1 (PARK7) mutations are less frequent than Parkin (PARK2) mutations in early-onset Parkinson disease. Neurology. 2004;62:389-94.

84. Bandopadhyay R, Kingsbury AE, Cookson MR, Reid AR, Evans IM, Hope AD, Pittman AM, Lashley T, Canet-Aviles R, Miller DW, McLendon C, Strand C, Leonard AJ, Abou-Sleiman PM, Healy DG, Ariga H, Wood NW, de Silva R, Revesz T, Hardy JA, Lees AJ. The expression of DJ-1 (PARK7) in normal human CNS and idiopathic Parkinson's disease. Brain. 2004;127:420-30.

85. Olzmann JA, Brown K, Wilkinson KD, Rees HD, Huai Q, Ke H, Levey AI, Li L, Chin LS. Familial Parkinson's disease-associated L166P mutation disrupts DJ-1 protein folding and function. J Biol Chem. 2004;279:8506-15.

86. Neumann M, Muller V, Gorner K, Kretzschmar HA, Haass C, Kahle PJ. Pathological properties of the Parkinson's disease-associated protein DJ-1 in alpha-synucleinopathies and tauopathies: relevance for multiple system atrophy and Pick's disease. Acta Neuropathol (Berl). 2004;107:489-96.

87. Rizzu P, Hinkle DA, Zhukareva V, Bonifati V, Severijnen LA, Martinez D, Ravid R, Kamphorst W, Eberwine JH, Lee VM, Trojanowski JQ, Heutink P. DJ-1 colocalizes with tau inclusions: a link between parkinsonism and dementia. Ann Neurol. 2004;55:113-8.

88. Morris HR. Genetics of Parkinson's disease. Ann Med. 2005;37:86-96.

89. Canet-Aviles RM, Wilson MA, Miller DW, Ahmad R, McLendon C, Bandyopadhyay S, Baptista MJ, Ringe D, Petsko GA, Cookson MR. The Parkinson's disease protein DJ-1 is neuroprotective due to cysteine-sulfinic acid-driven mitochondrial localization. Proc Natl Acad Sci U S A. 2004;101:9103-8.

90. Yokota T, Sugawara K, Ito K, Takahashi R, Ariga H, Mizusawa H. Down regulation of DJ-1 enhances cell death by oxidative stress, ER stress, and proteasome inhibition. Biochem Biophys Res Commun. 2003;312:1342-8.

91. Miller DW, Ahmad R, Hague S, Baptista MJ, Canet-Aviles R, McLendon C, Carter DM, Zhu PP, Stadler J, Chandran J, Klinefelter GR, Blackstone C, Cookson MR. L166P mutant DJ-1, causative for

recessive Parkinson's disease, is degraded through the ubiquitin-proteasome system. J Biol Chem. 2003;278:36588-95.

92. Taira T, Saito Y, Niki T, Iguchi-Ariga SM, Takahashi K, Ariga H. DJ-1 has a role in antioxidative stress to prevent cell death. EMBO Rep. 2004;5:213-8.

93. Moore DJ, Zhang L, Troncoso J, Lee MK, Hattori N, Mizuno Y, Dawson TM, Dawson VL. Association of DJ-1 and parkin mediated by pathogenic DJ-1 mutations and oxidative stress. Hum Mol Genet. 2005;14:71-84.

94. Funayama M, Hasegawa K, Kowa H, Saito M, Tsuji S, Obata F. A new locus for Parkinson's disease (PARK8) maps to chromosome 12p11.2-q13.1. Ann Neurol. 2002;51:296-301.

95. Deng H, Le W, Guo Y, Hunter CB, Xie W, Jankovic J. Genetic and clinical identification of Parkinson's disease patients with LRRK2 G2019S mutation. Ann Neurol. 2005;57:933-4.

96. Di Fonzo A, Rohe CF, Ferreira J, Chien HF, Vacca L, Stocchi F, Guedes L, Fabrizio E, Manfredi M, Vanacore N, Goldwurm S, Breedveld G, Sampaio C, Meco G, Barbosa E, Oostra BA, Bonifati V. A frequent LRRK2 gene mutation associated with autosomal dominant Parkinson's disease. Lancet. 2005;365:412-5.

97. Gilks WP, Abou-Sleiman PM, Gandhi S, Jain S, Singleton A, Lees AJ, Shaw K, Bhatia KP, Bonifati V, Quinn NP, Lynch J, Healy DG, Holton JL, Revesz T, Wood NW. A common LRRK2 mutation in idiopathic Parkinson's disease. Lancet. 2005;365:415-6.

98. Toft M, Mata IF, Kachergus JM, Ross OA, Farrer MJ. LRRK2 mutations and Parkinsonism. Lancet. 2005;365: 1229-30.

99. Paisan-Ruiz C, Jain S, Evans EW, Gilks WP, Simon J, van der Brug M, Lopez de Munain A, Aparicio S, Gil AM, Khan N, Johnson J, Martinez JR, Nicholl D, Carrera IM, Pena AS, de Silva R, Lees A, Marti-Masso JF, Perez-Tur J, Wood NW, Singleton AB. Cloning of the gene containing mutations that cause PARK8-linked Parkinson's disease. Neuron. 2004;44:595-600.

100. Aasly JO, Toft M, Fernandez-Mata I, Kachergus J, Hulihan M, White LR, Farrer M. Clinical features of LRRK2-associated Parkinson's disease in central Norway. Ann Neurol. 2005;57:762-5.

101. Kachergus J, Mata IF, Hulihan M, Taylor JP, Lincoln S, Aasly J, Gibson JM, Ross OA, Lynch T, Wiley J, Payami H, Nutt J, Maraganore DM, Czyzewski K, Styczynska M, Wszolek ZK, Farrer MJ, Toft M. Identification of a novel LRRK2 mutation linked to autosomal dominant parkinsonism: evidence of a common founder across European populations. Am J Hum Genet. 2005;76:672-80.

102. Foroud T. LRRK2: both a cause and a risk factor for Parkinson disease? Neurology. 2005;65:664-5.

103. Berg D, Schweitzer K, Leitner P, Zimprich A, Lichtner P, Belcredi P, Brussel T, Schulte C, Maass S, Nagele T. Type and frequency of mutations in the LRRK2 gene in familial and sporadic Parkinson's disease*. Brain. 2005;128:3000-11.

104. Lesage S, Ibanez P, Lohmann E, Pollak P, Tison F, Tazir M, Leutenegger AL, Guimaraes J, Bonnet AM, Agid Y, Durr A, Brice A. G2019S LRRK2 mutation in French and North African families with Parkinson's disease. Ann Neurol. 2005.58:784-7.

105. Wszolek ZK, Pfeiffer RF, Tsuboi Y, Uitti RJ, McComb RD, Stoessl AJ, Strongosky AJ, Zimprich A, Muller-Myhsok B, Farrer MJ, Gasser T, Calne DB, Dickson DW. Autosomal dominant parkinsonism associated with variable synuclein and tau pathology. Neurology. 2004;62:1619-22.

106. Zimprich A, Muller-Myhsok B, Farrer M, Leitner P, Sharma M, Hulihan M, Lockhart P, Strongosky A, Kachergus J, Calne DB, Stoessl J, Uitti RJ, Pfeiffer RF, Trenkwalder C, Homann N, Ott E, Wenzel K, Asmus F, Hardy J, Wszolek Z, Gasser T. The PARK8 locus in autosomal dominant parkinsonism: confirmation of linkage and further delineation of the disease-containing interval. Am J Hum Genet. 2004;74:11-9.

107. Scott WK, Grubber JM, Conneally PM, Small GW, Hulette CM, Rosenberg CK, Saunders AM, Roses AD, Haines JL, Pericak-Vance MA. Fine mapping of the chromosome 12 late-onset Alzheimer disease locus: potential genetic and phenotypic heterogeneity. Am J Hum Genet. 2000.66:922-32.

108. West AB, Zimprich A, Lockhart PJ, Farrer M, Singleton A, Holtom B, Lincoln S, Hofer A, Hill L, Muller-Myhsok B, Wszolek ZK, Hardy J, Gasser T. Refinement of the PARK3 locus on chromosome 2p13 and the analysis of 14 candidate genes. Eur J Hum Genet. 2001;9:659-66.

109. Karamohamed S, DeStefano AL, Wilk JB, Shoemaker CM, Golbe LI, Mark MH, Lazzarini AM, Suchowersky O, Labelle N, Guttman M, Currie LJ, Wooten GF, Stacy M, Saint-Hilaire M, Feldman RG, Sullivan KM, Xu G, Watts R, Growdon J, Lew M, Waters C, Vieregge P, Pramstaller PP, Klein C, Racette BA, Perlmutter JS, Parsian A, Singer C, Montgomery E, Baker K, Gusella JF, Fink SJ, Myers RH, Herbert A. A haplotype at the PARK3 locus influences onset age for Parkinson's disease: the GenePD study. Neurology. 2003;61:1557-61.

110. Hicks AA, Petursson H, Jonsson T, Stefansson H, Johannsdottir HS, Sainz J, Frigge ML, Kong A, Gulcher JR, Stefansson K,

Sveinbjornsdottir S. A susceptibility gene for late-onset idiopathic Parkinson's disease. Ann Neurol. 2002;52:549-55.

111. Pankratz N, Nichols WC, Uniacke SK, Halter C, Rudolph A, Shults C, Conneally PM, Foroud T. Significant linkage of Parkinson disease to chromosome 2q36-37. Am J Hum Genet. 2003;72:1053-7.

112. Le WD, Xu P, Jankovic J, Jiang H, Appel SH, Smith RG, Vassilatis DK. Mutations in NR4A2 associated with familial Parkinson disease. Nat Genet. 2003;33:85-9.

113. Hering R, Petrovic S, Mietz EM, Holzmann C, Berg D, Bauer P, Woitalla D, Muller T, Berger K, Kruger R, Riess O. Extended mutation analysis and association studies of Nurr1 (NR4A2) in Parkinson disease. Neurology. 2004;62:1231-2.

114. Zimprich A, Asmus F, Leitner P, Castro M, Bereznai B, Homann N, Ott E, Rutgers AW, Wieditz G, Trenkwalder C, Gasser T. Point mutations in exon 1 of the NR4A2 gene are not a major cause of familial Parkinson's disease. Neurogenetics. 2003;4:219-20.

115. Pankratz N, Nichols WC, Uniacke SK, Halter C, Rudolph A, Shults C, Conneally PM, Foroud T. Genome screen to identify susceptibility genes for Parkinson disease in a sample without parkin mutations. Am J Hum Genet. 2002;71:124-35.

116. Marx FP, Holzmann C, Strauss KM, Li L, Eberhardt O, Gerhardt E, Cookson MR, Hernandez D, Farrer MJ, Kachergus J, Engelender S, Ross CA, Berger K, Schols L, Schulz JB, Riess O, Kruger R. Identification and functional characterization of a novel R621C mutation in the synphilin-1 gene in Parkinson's disease. Hum Mol Genet. 2003;12:1223-31.

117. Mellick GD, Buchanan DD, McCann SJ, James KM, Johnson AG, Davis DR, Liyou N, Chan D, Le Couteur DG. Variations in the monoamine oxidase B (MAOB) gene are associated with Parkinson's disease. Mov Disord. 1999;14:219-24.

118. Nicholl DJ, Bennett P, Hiller L, Bonifati V, Vanacore N, Fabbrini G, Marconi R, Colosimo C, Lamberti P, Stocchi F, Bonuccelli U, Vieregge P, Ramsden DB, Meco G, Williams AC. A study of five candidate genes in Parkinson's disease and related neurodegenerative disorders. European Study Group on Atypical Parkinsonism. Neurology. 1999;53:1415-21.

119. Grevle L, Guzey C, Hadidi H, Brennersted R, Idle JR, Aasly J. Allelic association between the DRD2 TaqI A polymorphism and Parkinson's disease. Mov Disord. 2000;15:1070-4.

120. van der Walt JM, Nicodemus KK, Martin ER, Scott WK, Nance MA, Watts RL, Hubble JP, Haines JL, Koller WC, Lyons K, Pahwa R, Stern

MB, Colcher A, Hiner BC, Jankovic J, Ondo WG, Allen FH Jr, Goetz CG, Small GW, Mastaglia F, Stajich JM, McLaurin AC, Middleton LT, Scott BL, Schmechel DE, Pericak-Vance MA, Vance JM. Mitochondrial polymorphisms significantly reduce the risk of Parkinson disease. Am J Hum Genet. 2003;72:804-11.

121. Aarsland D, Andersen K, Larsen JP, Lolk A, Kragh-Sorensen P. Prevalence and characteristics of dementia in Parkinson disease: an 8-year prospective study. Arch Neurol. 2003;60:387-92.

122. de Lau LM, Schipper CM, Hofman A, Koudstaal PJ, Breteler MM. Prognosis of Parkinson disease: risk of dementia and mortality: the Rotterdam Study. Arch Neurol. 2005;62:1265-9.

123. McKeith IG, Dickson DW, Lowe J, Emre M, O'Brien JT, Feldman H, Cummings J, Duda JE, Lippa C, Perry EK, Aarsland D, Arai H, Ballard CG, Boeve B, Burn DJ, Costa D, Del Ser T, Dubois B, Galasko D, Gauthier S, Goetz CG, Gomez-Tortosa E, Halliday G, Hansen LA, Hardy J, Iwatsubo T, Kalaria RN, Kaufer D, Kenny RA, Korczyn A, Kosaka K, Lee VM, Lees A, Litvan I, Londos E, Lopez OL, Minoshima S, Mizuno Y, Molina JA, Mukaetova-Ladinska EB, Pasquier F, Perry RH, Schulz JB, Trojanowski JQ, Yamada M. Diagnosis and management of dementia with Lewy bodies: third report of the DLB Consortium. Neurology. 2005;65:1863-72.

124. Kurz MW, Schlitter AM, Larsen JP, Ballard C, Aarsland D. Familial occurrence of dementia and parkinsonism: a systematic review. Dement Geriatr Cogn Disord. 2006;22:288-95.

125. Waters CH, Miller CA. Autosomal dominant Lewy body parkinsonism in a four-generation family. Ann Neurol. 1994;35:59-64.

126. Aarsland D, Perry R, Brown A, Larsen JP, Ballard C. Neuropathology of dementia in Parkinson's disease: a prospective, community-based study. Ann Neurol. 2005;58:773-6.

127. Johnson J, Hague SM, Hanson M, Gibson A, Wilson KE, Evans EW, Singleton AA, McInerney-Leo A, Nussbaum RL, Hernandez DG, Gallardo M, McKeith IG, Burn DJ, Ryu M, Hellstrom O, Ravina B, Eerola J, Perry RH, Jaros E, Tienari P, Weiser R, Gwinn-Hardy K, Morris CM, Hardy J, Singleton AB. SNCA multiplication is not a common cause of Parkinson disease or dementia with Lewy bodies. Neurology. 2004;63:554-6.

128. Mahley RW, Rall SC Jr. Apolipoprotein E: far more than a lipid transport protein. Annu Rev Genomics Hum Genet. 2000;1:507-37.

129. Houlston RS, Snowden C, Green F, Alberti KG, Humphries SE. Apolipoprotein (apo) E genotypes by polymerase chain reaction and allele-specific oligonucleotide probes: no detectable linkage

disequilibrium between apo E and apo CII. Hum Genet. 1989;83:364-8.

130. Feussner G, Feussner V, Hoffmann MM, Lohrmann J, Wieland H, Marz W. Molecular basis of type III hyperlipoproteinemia in Germany. Hum Mutat. 1998;11:417-23.

131. DeKroon RM, Mihovilovic M, Goodger ZV, Robinette JB, Sullivan PM, Saunders AM, Strittmatter WJ. ApoE genotype-specific inhibition of apoptosis. J Lipid Res. 2003;44:1566-73.

132. Strittmatter WJ, Saunders AM, Schmechel D, Pericak-Vance M, Enghild J, Salvesen GS, Roses AD. Apolipoprotein E: high-avidity binding to beta-amyloid and increased frequency of type 4 allele in late-onset familial Alzheimer disease. Proc Natl Acad Sci U S A. 1993;90:1977-81.

133. Mayeux R. Gene-environment interaction in late-onset Alzheimer disease: the role of apolipoprotein-epsilon4. Alzheimer Dis Assoc Disord. 1998;12 Suppl 3:S10-5.

134. Lopez OL, Lopez-Pousa S, Kamboh MI, Adroer R, Oliva R, Lozano-Gallego M, Becker JT, DeKosky ST. Apolipoprotein E polymorphism in Alzheimer's disease: a comparative study of two research populations from Spain and the United States. Eur Neurol. 1998;39:229-33.

135. Harhangi BS, de Rijk MC, van Duijn CM, Van Broeckhoven C, Hofman A, Breteler MM. APOE and the risk of PD with or without dementia in a population-based study. Neurology. 2000;54:1272-6.

136. Huang X, Chen PC, Poole C. APOE-[varepsilon]2 allele associated with higher prevalence of sporadic Parkinson disease. Neurology. 2004;62:2198-202.

137. Inzelberg R, Paleacu D, Chapman J, Korczyn AD. Apolipoprotein E and Parkinson's disease. Ann Neurol. 1998;44:294; author reply 295.

138. Li YJ, Hauser MA, Scott WK, Martin ER, Booze MW, Qin XJ, Walter JW, Nance MA, Hubble JP, Koller WC, Pahwa R, Stern MB, Hiner BC, Jankovic J, Goetz CG, Small GW, Mastaglia F, Haines JL, Pericak-Vance MA, Vance JM. Apolipoprotein E controls the risk and age at onset of Parkinson disease. Neurology. 2004;62:2005-9.

139. Parsian A, Racette B, Goldsmith LJ, Perlmutter JS. Parkinson's disease and apolipoprotein E: possible association with dementia but not age at onset. Genomics. 2002;79:458-61.

140. Huang X, Chen P, Kaufer DI, Troster AI, Poole C. Apolipoprotein E and dementia in Parkinson disease: a meta-analysis. Arch Neurol. 2006;63:189-93.

141. de la Fuente-Fernandez R, Nunez MA, Lopez E. The apolipoprotein E epsilon 4 allele increases the risk of drug-induced hallucinations in Parkinson's disease. Clin Neuropharmacol. 1999;22:226-30.

142. Oliveri RL, Nicoletti G, Cittadella R, Manna I, Branca D, Zappia M, Gambardella A, Caracciolo M, Quattrone A. Apolipoprotein E polymorphisms and Parkinson's disease. Neurosci Lett. 1999;277:83-6.

143. Goetz CG, Burke PF, Leurgans S, Berry-Kravis E, Blasucci LM, Raman R, Zhou L. Genetic variation analysis in parkinson disease patients with and without hallucinations: case-control study. Arch Neurol. 2001;58:209-13.

144. Zareparsi S, Kaye J, Camicioli R, Grimslid H, Oken B, Litt M, Nutt J, Bird T, Schellenberg G, Payami H. Modulation of the age at onset of Parkinson's disease by apolipoprotein E genotypes. Ann Neurol. 1997;42:655-8.

145. Pankratz N, Byder L, Halter C, Rudolph A, Shults CW, Conneally PM, Foroud T, Nichols WC. Presence of an APOE4 allele results in significantly earlier onset of Parkinson's disease and a higher risk with dementia. Mov Disord. 2006;21:45-9.

146. Maraganore DM, Farrer MJ, Hardy JA, McDonnell SK, Schaid DJ, Rocca WA. Case-control study of debrisoquine 4-hydroxylase, N-acetyltransferase 2, and apolipoprotein E gene polymorphisms in Parkinson's disease. Mov Disord. 2000;15:714-9.

147. Kurosinski P, Guggisberg M, Gotz J. Alzheimer's and Parkinson's disease--overlapping or synergistic pathologies? Trends Mol Med. 2002;8:3-5.

148. Li YJ, Pericak-Vance MA, Haines JL, Siddique N, McKenna-Yasek D, Hung WY, Sapp P, Allen CI, Chen W, Hosler B, Saunders AM, Dellefave LM, Brown RH, Siddique T. Apolipoprotein E is associated with age at onset of amyotrophic lateral sclerosis. Neurogenetics. 2004;5:209-13.

149. Schmidt S, Klaver C, Saunders A, Postel E, De La Paz M, Agarwal A, Small K, Udar N, Ong J, Chalukya M, Nesburn A, Kenney C, Domurath R, Hogan M, Mah T, Conley Y, Ferrell R, Weeks D, de Jong PT, van Duijn C, Haines J, Pericak-Vance M, Gorin M. A pooled case-control study of the apolipoprotein E (APOE) gene in age-related maculopathy. Ophthalmic Genet. 2002;23:209-23.

150. Kurz MW, Larsen JP, Kvaloy JT, Aarsland D. Associations between family history of Parkinson's disease and dementia and risk of dementia in Parkinson's disease: a community-based, longitudinal study. Mov Disord. 2006;21:2170-4.

151. Zimprich A, Biskup S, Leitner P, Lichtner P, Farrer M, Lincoln S, Kachergus J, Hulihan M, Uitti RJ, Calne DB, Stoessl AJ, Pfeiffer RF, Patenge N, Carbajal IC, Vieregge P, Asmus F, Muller-Myhsok B, Dickson DW, Meitinger T, Strom TM, Wszolek ZK, Gasser T. Mutations in LRRK2 cause autosomal-dominant parkinsonism with pleomorphic pathology. Neuron. 2004;44:601-7.

4

The Role of the Ubiquitin-Proteasome System in Parkinson's Disease

Kevin St. P. McNaught[1], Nicholas MacInnes[2], and Peter Jenner[2]

[1]Mount Sinai School of Medicine;
[2]King's College London.

Address correspondence to Dr. Kevin McNaught, Department of Neurology, Mount Sinai School of Medicine, Annenberg 14-73, One Gustave L. Levy Place, New York, NY 10029. Tel: 212-241-4251; Fax: 212-987-0348.
E-mail: kevin.mcnaught@mssm.edu

Acknowledgments: This study was supported by grants from the Bachmann-Strauss Dystonia & Parkinson Foundation Inc., the Bendheim Parkinson's Disease Center, the Schapiro Foundation, and the NIH/NINDS (1 RO1 NS045999-01).

OUTLINE

Introduction
Protein Handling in the Central Nervous System
Parkin Mutations
UCH-L1
α-Synuclein
DJ-1
PINK1
LRRK2/Dardarin
Sporadic Parkinson's Disease: Altered Proteasomal Function
    Proteasomal Dysfunction
    Role of Proteasomal Dysfunction
    Cause of Proteasomal Dysfunction
    Relationship between the UPS and Other Biochemical
    Changes in Parkinson's Disease
    Role of Proteasomal Dysfunction in Lewy Body
    Formation
    The Role of the Proteasome in the Age-Related
    Susceptibility of the SNc
Conclusion
References

INTRODUCTION

Parkinson's disease is a slowly progressive, neurological disorder that typically manifests during mid to late life[1,2]. The illness affects males and females, occurs in all races/ethnic groups, and is seen worldwide with some variations in incidence/prevalence rates[3]. Parkinson's disease is characterized pathologically by a loss of melanized dopaminergic neurons in the substantia nigra pars compacta (SNc), resulting in the depletion of dopamine content in the striatum[4]. Neurodegeneration with loss of neurotransmitters can also occur in other brain regions, in particular the locus ceruleus (LC), dorsal motor nucleus of the vagus (DMN), nucleus basalis of Meynert (NBM), and olfactory system[4–6], as well as in peripheral autonomic ganglia (e.g., superior cervical ganglion and mesenteric plexus)[7]. Characteristically, neuronal degeneration is accompanied by intracytoplasmic, proteinaceous inclusions known as Lewy bodies at the various pathological sites[4,5,8].

The etiology of Parkinson's disease is not known in the large majority of cases. Approximately 10–15% of cases are thought to be genetic in origin and, currently, 11 different linkages with six identified gene mutations have been discovered in small numbers of familial cases of the disorder (Table 1)[9–11]. Most cases (approximately 90%) of Parkinson's disease occur sporadically and are of unknown cause. Epidemiologic studies suggest that environmental factors play an important role in these patients, who may be rendered susceptible by their genetic profile, poor ability to metabolize toxins, and/or advancing age[12]. The specific environmental agent/toxin has not been identified, although several candidates have been suggested, and it appears likely that a different combination of environmental and genetic factors may be responsible for the disorder in different patients or subtypes of Parkinson's disease.

The pathogenic mechanism responsible for neurodegeneration in Parkinson's disease is not established, although it is thought to occur by way of a signal-mediated, apoptotic process[13] and to involve a cascade of events that include oxidative stress[14], mitochondrial dysfunction[15], inflammation[16], and excitotoxicity[17].

Table 1. Implication of the UPS in Familial and Sporadic Parkinson's Disease

Locus	Chromosome Location	Gene Product and Properties	Mutations	Inheritance Pattern
PARK 1 and 4	4q21-q23	α-Synuclein	Point mutations (A53T, A30P, and E46K)	Autosomal dominant
		140-amino-acid/ 14-kDa protein	Duplication	
		Localized to synaptic terminals	Triplication	
		Function: unknown; possibly play a role in synaptic activity		
PARK 2	6q25.2-q27	Parkin	Deletions	Autosomal recessive
		465-amino-acid/ 52-kDa protein	Point mutations	Rarely autosomal dominant
		Expressed in cytoplasm, Golgi complex, nuclei, and processes	Multiplications	
		Function: E3 ubiquitin ligase		
PARK 5	4p14	UCH-L1	Missense mutation (I93M)	Autosomal dominant
		230-amino-acid/ 26-kDa protein		
		Neuron-specific protein		
		Function: deubiquitinating enzyme (possible E3 activity also)		
PARK 6	1p35-1p36	PINK 1	Missense	AR
		581-amino-acid/ 62.8-kDa protein	Truncating	
		Localized to mitochondria		
		Function: unknown; may be a protein kinase		
PARK 7	1p36	DJ-1	Deletion	AR
		189-amino-acid/ 20-kDa protein	Truncating	
		More prominent in the cytoplasm and nucleus of astrocytes compared to neurons	Missense	
		Function: unknown; possible antioxidant, molecular chaperone, and protease		
PARK 8	12p11.2-12q31.1	Dardarin/LRRK2	Missense	AD
		2482/2527 amino acids		
		Function: unknown; may be a protein kinase		
Sporadic Parkinson's disease	—		—	—

Table 1 (continued)

Locus	Age of Onset (Year)	Clinical Spectrum	Pathological Features	Possible (Theoretical) Basis for Altered Protein Handling
PARK 1 and 4	Range: 30–60 Mean: 45	Levodopa-responsive; rapid progression; prominent dementia	Neuronal loss in the SNc, LC, and DMN	α-Synuclein is prone to misfold and mutations enhance this property.
		E46K and multiplication cases demonstrate overlap with DLB	Lewy bodies are rare and tau accumulation occurs in some A53T cases; extensive Lewy bodies in E46K and multiplication cases.	Mutations/over-production of α-synuclein could lead to a cycle of events that include α-synuclein misfolding, aggregation, proteasomal dysfunction, generalized protein aggregation, and neurodegeneration.
			Triplication cases demonstrate degeneration in the hippocampus, vacuolization in the cortex, and glial cytoplasmic inclusions.	
PARK 2	Range: 7–58 Mean: 26.1	Levodopa-responsive and severe dyskinesias; foot dystonia; diurnal fluctuations; hyperreflexia; slow progression	Selective and severe destruction of the SNc and LC	Parkin is a ubiquitin ligase.
			Generally Lewy body negative	Parkin mutations could impair ubiquitination of target proteins, which might then accumulate, aggregate, and cause cell death.
PARK 5	49 and 50	Typical Parkinson's disease	Lewy bodies reported in a single case	UCH-L1 is a deubiquitinating enzyme. Failure to deubiquitinate might prevent ubiquitinated proteins from being able to enter the proteasome and be degraded.

Table 1 (continued)

Locus	Age of Onset (Year)	Clinical Spectrum	Pathological Features	Possible (Theoretical) Basis for Altered Protein Handling
				It might also limit the supply of ubiquitin monomers necessary for the clearance of additional unwanted proteins.
PARK 6	Range: 32–48	Levodopa-responsive; slow progression	Neuropathology not yet determined	PINK1 prevents proteasome inhibitor–induced mitochondrial dysfunction and cell death, but protection is lost with mutations found in Parkinson's disease. Mutations in PINK1 could render neurons vulnerable to toxins that act as proteasome inhibitors. PINK1 mutations could also impair mitochondrial function.
PARK 7	Range: 20–40s Mean: mid 30s	Levodopa responsive; dystonia; psychiatric disturbance; slow progression	Neuropathology not yet determined	Antioxidant or sensor of oxidative stress; molecular structure suggests that it has molecular chaperone and protease activity; interacts with parkin and CHIP/HSP70 Mutations as in Parkinson's disease destabilize DJ-1 and inactivate its proteolytic activity. Overexpression protects cultured cells from oxidative stress, while knockdown increases susceptibility to oxidative stress, endoplasmic reticulum stress, and proteasomal inhibition. Wild-type DJ-1 inhibits aggregation of α-synuclein, and effect is lost when DJ-1 is mutated as in Parkinson's disease.

Table 1 (continued)

Locus	Age of Onset (Year)	Clinical Spectrum	Pathological Features	Possible (Theoretical) Basis for Altered Protein Handling
PARK 8	Range: 35–79 Mean: 57.4	Typical Parkinson's disease features; slow progression; dementia present; features of motor neuron disease reported	SNc degeneration	Sequence suggests that the mutation might lead to increased kinase activity, which could promote altered phosphorylation and misfolding of substrates.
			Some cases show extensive Lewy bodies; some do not have Lewy bodies	
			Also, intranuclear inclusions, tau-immunoreactive inclusions, and neurofibrillary tangles are present	
Sporadic Parkinson's disease	Mean: approx. 60 years	Levodopa responsive	Degeneration in SNc with Lewy bodies	Reduced α-subunits of 20S proteasome
		Resting tremor, rigidity, bradykinesia, gait dysfunction, asymmetry	Degeneration with Lewy bodies in selected additional locations involving neurons of LC, NBM, DMV, olfactory, autonomic system.	Reduced proteasomal enzyme activity
		Gradually progressive		Reduced compensatory responses in proteasome activators

More recently, genetic, postmortem, and experimental evidence have converged to suggest that a failure of the ubiquitin-proteasome system (UPS) to degrade misfolded proteins plays a major role in the etiopathogenesis of some familial and sporadic forms of Parkinson's disease[9,11,18] (Figure 1). In this chapter, we will examine these findings and consider how alterations in UPS function might play a role in the etiology and pathogenesis of Parkinson's disease.

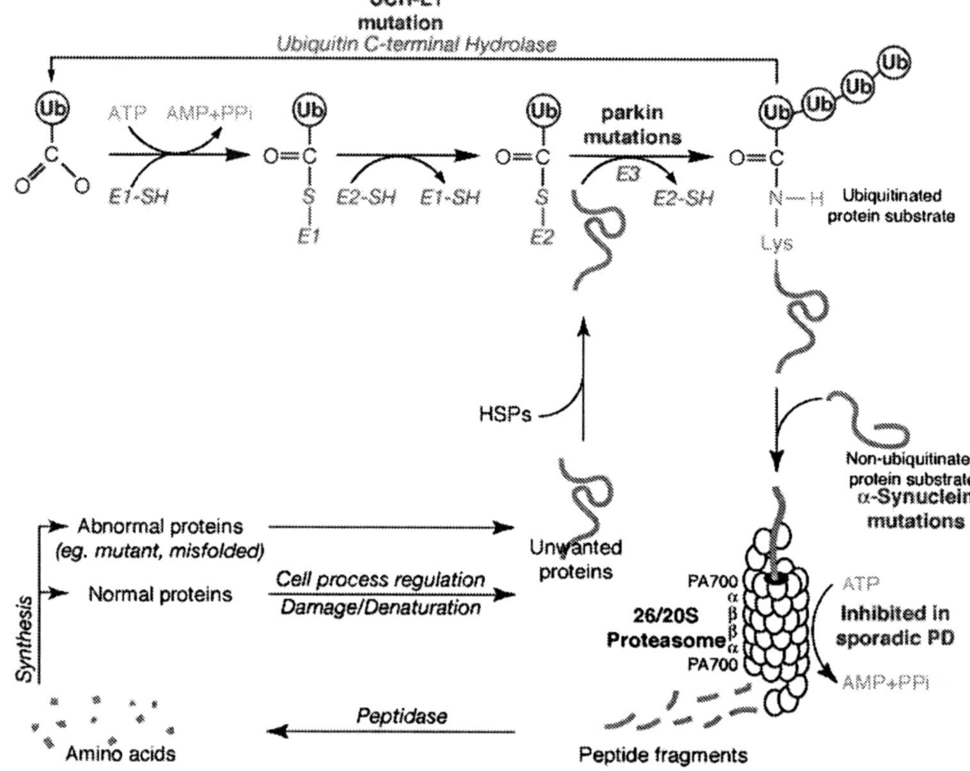

FIGURE 1. The UPS and Parkinson's disease.

PROTEIN HANDLING IN THE CENTRAL NERVOUS SYSTEM

The UPS is the major pathway for mediating the degradation of unwanted, intracellular, soluble proteins (i.e., mutant, misfolded, denatured, misplaced, or damaged proteins) in the cytoplasm, nucleus, and endoplasmic reticulum of eukaryocytic cells[19–22]. The process whereby the UPS clears these unwanted proteins typically involves the following sequence: (a) ATP-dependent activation of ubiquitin monomers, (b) labeling of unwanted/damaged proteins with chains of activated ubiquitin molecules, (c) transport of ubiquitinated proteins to the proteasome by chaperone molecules (e.g., heat shock proteins), (d) the recognition and unfolding of ubiquitinated proteins by proteasomal regulators, and finally (e) ATP-dependent degradation of the protein by the 26/20S proteasome[19–22]. Proteasomal degradation of proteins yields short peptide fragments (2–25 residues) that are further degraded by peptidases into their constituent amino acids, which can then be recycled into new proteins[23]. Prior to entry into the proteasome, ubiquitin chains are detached from protein conjugates by deubiquitinating enzymes (ubiquitin C-terminal hydrolases) and disassembled into monomeric ubiquitin molecules that can be recycled to facilitate the clearance of additional unwanted proteins.

Some proteins (e.g., oxidatively damaged proteins) can be directly degraded by the 20S proteasome (the catalytic core of the 26S proteasome) in an ATP-independent manner and without prior ubiquitination[24]. Proteins that are excessively misfolded or aggregated can resist degradation and even inhibit proteasomal function, possibly by blocking the inner chamber of the proteasome[25,26]. Heat shock proteins (HSPs), such as HSP70 and HSP90, play an important role in protein handling. They up-regulate in the presence of excess levels of misfolded proteins and promote the refolding of proteins to their native state. They also act as chaperones to transport abnormal proteins to the proteasome for degradation[21,27,28].

Cells normally maintain a dynamic balance between the generation and clearance of unwanted proteins. Disturbance of this equilibrium, either by excess formation of unwanted proteins or by impaired protein degradation, leads to an adverse state called proteolytic stress[11,29]. Under these circumstances, undegraded proteins accumulate and aggregate with each other, as well as with normal proteins. Protein aggregates can impair UPS function[21,24,30], interfere with intracellular processes (e.g., axonal transport, synaptic plasticity, and neurotransmission), inactivate HSPs, and induce cytotoxicity[24,31–34].

There is abundant evidence from genetic, pathologic, and experimental studies that suggests that the pathogenesis of some familial and sporadic forms of Parkinson's disease may be related to a defect in the capacity of the UPS (Figure 1).

PARKIN MUTATIONS

In 1973, an early-onset form of autosomal-recessive Parkinson's disease was recognized in Japanese families (AR-JP)[35] and linked to chromosome 6q25.2-q27 (PARK 2)[35,36]. The gene encodes a 465-

amino-acid/52-kDa protein called parkin[37,38]. It is now known that parkin is a ubiquitin ligase that attaches ubiquitin molecules to substrate proteins[39–43]. Several deletions, multiplications, and point mutations in this gene have been identified[9], and it has been estimated that parkin mutations could be responsible for as much as 50% of early-onset cases[44].

The clinical features of AR-JP vary from sporadic Parkinson's disease in that there is an early age of onset (average 26.1 years) and a slow rate of disease progression[44]. Patients are characterized by foot dystonia at disease onset, diurnal fluctuations, hyperreflexia, transient improvement in motor disability after rest, infrequent rest tremor, a dramatic response to levodopa, and a propensity to develop dyskinesias[44]. Pathology in AR-JP also differs from sporadic Parkinson's disease in that neurodegeneration is confined to the SNc and LC, and Lewy bodies are typically absent[45]. Some late-onset cases with a parkin mutation have been described with a more typical Parkinson's disease picture[46] and Lewy bodies at postmortem[47].

Parkin is expressed in the cytoplasm, nucleus, Golgi apparatus, and processes of neurons[48]. Similar to other ubiquitin ligases, parkin has a modular structure containing a ubiquitin-like (UBL) domain at the N-terminus, a central linker region, and a RING finger domain at the C-terminus. Parkin acts in conjunction with the E2 enzymes Ubc6, UbcH7, and UbcH8 to ubiquitinate a variety of substrates, which are thought to include synphilin-1, CDCrel-1, parkin-associated endothelin-like receptor (Pael-R), O-glycosylated isoform of α-synuclein (αSp22), cyclin E α/β-tubulin, p38 subunit of aminoacyl-tRNA synthetase complex, and synaptotagmin X1[9,39,41,42]. Parkin, through its UBL domain, interacts with the 26S proteasome subunit Rpn10/S5a that, along with the Rpt5/S6′ subunit, plays a role in the recognition of ubiquitinated substrates by the PA700 regulatory cap[20,49]. Parkin also binds to the HSP complex CHIP/HSP70 and may promote its activity[50,51].

The mechanism by which mutations in parkin induce neurodegeneration is not firmly established, but likely relates to a loss of ubiquitin ligase activity and a reduced capacity to label substrate proteins for proteasomal degradation. In support of this concept, patients with AR-JP have markedly reduced parkin protein and enzyme activity in areas that degenerate (SNc and LC)[39,40,45,52], and there is an accumulation of nonubiquitinated parkin substrates (Pael-R, αSp22) in these regions[40,42]. This concept is further supported by the demonstration that parkin protein prevents cell death induced by overexpression of Pael-R in both cultured cells and *Drosophila*[41,42,53]. Thus, parkin mutations could impair ubiquitination and degradation of target proteins that might then accumulate, aggregate, and cause cell death. Interestingly, parkin also protects against cell death induced by overexpression of α-synuclein even though this is not thought to be a parkin substrate, suggesting that parkin might act through other mechanisms, such as enhanced chaperone function[54].

It is interesting that neither transgenic mice that express parkin mutations nor parkin knockout mice develop nigrostriatal degeneration[55–59]. Further, the frequency of parkin point mutations is similar in Parkinson's disease patients (3.8%) and control subjects (3.1%)[60]. These observations raise the possibility that patients with parkin mutations may require other factors, such as additional genetic alterations or exposure to environmental toxins, to trigger neurodegeneration and the development of parkinsonism.

UCH-L1

In 1998, Leroy and colleagues reported that an I93M missense mutation in the gene (4p14; PARK 5) that encodes ubiquitin C-terminal L1 (UCH-L1) was identified in association with a Parkinson's disease syndrome in two German siblings[61]. The affected patients had a clinical picture that closely resembled sporadic Parkinson's disease, including a good response to levodopa, but symptoms emerged at a relatively early age (49 and 51 years). Postmortem study in one noted the presence of Lewy bodies[62]. Genetic screening has failed to detect UCH-L1 mutations in other Parkinson's disease patients[63], suggesting that this mutation must be a rare cause of Parkinson's disease. However, there is evidence that the UCH-L1 gene is a susceptibility locus and that polymorphisms, particularly the S18Y substitution, confer some degree of protection against developing the illness[64]. It is noteworthy, however, that a more recent study failed to show any association between the SY18 polymorphism in UCH-L1 and protection against developing Parkinson's disease[65].

UCH-L1 is a 230-amino-acid/26-kDa protein. It is expressed exclusively in neurons in many areas of the central nervous system (CNS)[66] and is thought to constitute 1–2% of soluble proteins in the brain[66–68]. UCH-L1 is a deubiquitinating enzyme that removes ubiquitin from protein adducts prior to their entry into the proteasome. UCH-L1 may also have ubiquitin ligase activity and plays a role in targeting proteins for proteasomal degradation[69]. Toxins that act on UCH-L1 cause a reduction in deubiquitinating activity and reduced ubiquitin levels *in vitro*[61,70,71]. Inhibition of ubiquitin C-terminal hydrolases in rat ventral midbrain cell cultures leads to degeneration of dopaminergic neurons with the formation of Lewy body–like inclusions[72]. In mice with a mutation in UCH-L1 (gracile axonal dystrophy), there is a reduction in deubiquitinating activity, formation of neuronal inclusions, and development of cerebellar degeneration, but it is unclear if these animals develop nigrostriatal pathology[71,73]. In Parkinson's disease patients with UCH-L1 mutation, it can be hypothesized that failure to deubiquitinate might prevent ubiquitinated proteins from being able to enter the proteasome and reduce the supply of ubiquitin monomers necessary for the clearance of additional unwanted proteins.

α-SYNUCLEIN

In 1996, the first gene identified in association with hereditary Parkinson's disease was linked to chromosome 4q21-q23 (PARK 1) in a large Italian family (the Contursi kindred). The illness was transmitted in an autosomal-dominant manner (full penetrance) and affected approximately 60 individuals spanning five generations[74,75]. It was subsequently determined that the responsible defect was an A53T mutation in the gene that encodes for α-synuclein, a 140-amino-acid/14-kDa protein of unknown function[76]. This mutation and inheritance pattern was also found in several unrelated Greek families[76]. In addition, Parkinson's disease syndromes have been associated with an A30P mutation in a German family (autosomal-dominant, reduced penetrance)[77] and with an E46K mutation in a Spanish family[78]. More recently, Parkinson's disease has been described in patients with duplication (in French and Italian families)[79,80] and triplication (Iowan kindred of mixed northern European origin and a Swedish-American family)[81–84] of the normal α-synuclein gene.

The clinical characteristics of Parkinson's disease linked to α-synuclein mutations share similarities with sporadic Parkinson's disease, but there is a relatively early age of onset (mean of approximately 40 years) and a high occurrence of dementia. Indeed, some of the patients with multiplication of the normal α-synuclein gene present with a clinical picture suggestive of dementia with Lewy bodies (DLB)[79–84]. Pathologically, patients with the A53T mutation showed a marked increase in α-synuclein–positive protein aggregates in various brain regions, but Lewy bodies are rare, and there was prominent accumulation of α-synuclein and tau in the cerebral cortex and striatum[82,85,86]. Patients with triplication of the α-synuclein gene had vacuolization in the cortex, neurodegeneration in the hippocampus, and glial cytoplasmic inclusions, which are not features of sporadic Parkinson's disease[82].

α-Synuclein, so called because of its localization to synapses and the nuclear envelope[87,88], belongs to a family of related proteins that include β- and γ-synucleins[89]. α-Synuclein is expressed throughout the CNS and is enriched in presynaptic terminals, lipid membranes, and vesicles[66,89]. The function of α-synuclein is unknown, but it is thought to play a role in synaptic neurotransmission and plasticity[89,90], but knockout of α-synuclein is not associated with synaptic change, neurodegeneration, or Parkinson's disease–like behavior[91].

Since the discovery of α-synuclein–linked familial Parkinson's disease, there has been a great deal of effort aimed at deciphering how mutations in the protein induce neurodegeneration. The dominant mode of inheritance suggests a gain of function. Wild-type α-synuclein is monomeric and intrinsically unstructured/natively unfolded at low concentrations, but in high concentration, it has a propensity to aggregate and oligomerize into β-pleated sheets[92,93]. Mutations in the protein increase this potential for misfolding, oligomerization, and aggregation[92,94–97]. Oligomerization of α-synuclein produces intermediary species (protofibrils) that form annular structures with pore-like properties that permeabilize synthetic vesicular membranes[94–96]. It has been suggested that protofibrils are the toxic α-synuclein species responsible for Lewy body formation and cell death[97], but this concept is largely based on studies of the biophysical and conformational properties of α-synuclein *in vitro*.

There are several reasons to consider that cell death associated with α-synuclein mutations/overproduction could involve defective clearance of the protein by the proteasome. Wild-type α-synuclein is a substrate for both the 26S and 20S proteasome, and is preferentially degraded in a ubiquitin-independent manner[98–100]. *In vitro* and *in vivo* studies have demonstrated that mutant α-synuclein resists proteasomal degradation and inhibits proteasomal function[101–103], which may account for why mutations in α-synuclein are associated with the accumulation of a wide range of intracellular proteins. Further, high levels of undegraded or poorly degraded normal α-synuclein protein have a tendency to self-aggregate, induce aggregation of other proteins, interfere with intracellular functions, and induce cytotoxicity[31]. Interestingly, recent studies indicate that α-synuclein can be broken down by the 20S proteasome through endoproteolytic degradation that does not involve the N- or C-terminus[98–100]. This type of degradation yields truncated α-synuclein fragments, which are particularly prone to aggregate and promote aggregation of the full-length protein[104]. Thus, it is possible that mutations/overproduction of α-synuclein could lead to a cycle of events that include α-synuclein misfolding, aggregation, proteasomal dysfunction, generalized protein aggregation, and neurodegeneration.

There have been many studies that examined the effects of α-synuclein mutations/overexpression in *in vitro* and transgenic animal models[105]. Overexpression of mutant α-synuclein can induce degeneration of dopaminergic neurons and accelerate cell death induced by other toxins[106]. Overexpression of mutant (A53T, A30P) or wild-type α-synuclein in *Drosophila* results in motor impairment, loss of SNc dopamine neurons, and inclusion body formation[107]. Similarly, SNc dopamine cell loss occurs following adenovirus delivery of A53T mutant or wild-type α-synuclein into the SNc of common marmosets[108]. However, overexpression of wild-type or mutant α-synuclein does not lead to neurodegeneration or parkinsonism in transgenic mice[105]. This observation may relate to findings that normal α-synuclein in some animal species has a threonine in the alanine position, as is found with the human mutation[76], or α-synuclein may be degraded differently in this species. Alternatively, it could be that additional factors, such as gene changes or toxins in the environment, might be required to trigger neurodegeneration in mice and humans. Indeed, not all carriers of point mutations in α-synuclein develop Parkinson's disease.

α-Synuclein can also be degraded by the lysosomal system and there is evidence of impaired clearance by autophagy of the mutant form of the protein[109,110]. The relative roles of the UPS and lysosomal systems in the degradation of wild-type and mutant α-synuclein has not yet been clearly defined, and it is possible that defects in the lysosomal systems could contribute to the protein accumulation and aggregation found in α-synuclein–linked familial Parkinson's disease.

DJ-1

In 2001, an autosomal-recessive, early-onset form of parkinsonism was described in Italian and Dutch families linked to a mutation in chromosome 1p36 (PARK 7)[111]. Parkinson's disease in these patients is related to deletion, truncating, and missense mutations in the gene that encodes the 189-amino-acid/20-kDa protein (DJ-1)[112–114]. It is estimated that these mutations account for 1–2% of early-onset

Parkinson's disease cases[115]. The clinical picture is characterized by early onset (mid 30s), slow progression, dystonia, good levodopa response, and psychiatric disturbances[112,113]. The neuropathological features of patients with DJ-1 mutations have not yet been reported.

DJ-1 is widely expressed in the CNS, is more prominent in astrocytes than neurons, and is present in the cytosol and nucleus of cells[116,117]. The function of DJ-1 is unknown, but there is evidence to suggest that it acts as an antioxidant or a sensor of oxidative stress[118,119]. In addition, its molecular structure and *in vitro* properties suggest that it has molecular chaperone and protease activity[120–122]. DJ-1 has also been shown to interact with parkin and CHIP/HSP70, suggesting a possible link to these proteolytic systems[123]. The mechanism whereby mutant DJ-1 induces cell death in Parkinson's disease is unknown, but the recessive pattern of inheritance raises the possibility of a loss of function of the mutant protein. Mutations as occur in Parkinson's disease (e.g., L166P) destabilize DJ-1, inactivate and impair its proteolytic activity, and promote its rapid degradation by the proteasome[120,124]. Overexpression of DJ-1 protects cultured cells from oxidative stress, while knockdown of DJ-1 increases susceptibility to oxidative stress, endoplasmic reticulum stress, and proteasomal inhibition[118,119]. Importantly, wild-type DJ-1 inhibits the aggregation of α-synuclein, but this effect is lost when DJ-1 is mutated as in Parkinson's disease[125]. Deletion of DJ-1 in transgenic mice does not induce neurodegeneration[126], suggesting that, here too, other factors might be involved in the pathogenic process in Parkinson's disease. These findings raise the possibility that a mutation in DJ-1 could be linked to a defect in UPS function by promoting protein aggregation and limiting protein clearance, although no evidence of proteolytic stress has been observed in transgenic mice with a deletion of DJ-1[126].

PINK1

Several European families with autosomal-recessive, early-onset Parkinson's disease were found to have missense and truncating mutations in a gene located at chromosome 1p35 (PARK 6), which encodes for a protein designated as PINK1 (PTEN [phosphatase and tensin homolog deleted on chromosome 10]-induced kinase 1)[127–129]. Subsequent studies found other affected families with this mutation[130]. The clinical expression of Parkinson's disease in patients with this mutation is characterized by early onset (32–48 years of age), slow progression, and a good response to levodopa[127,130].

PINK1 is a 581-amino-acid/62.8-kDa protein that is localized to mitochondria[129]. The normal function of PINK1 is unknown, but its structure suggests that it might be a serine/threonine protein kinase that phosphorylates proteins involved in signal transduction pathways[129]. In cultured cells, wild-type PINK1 prevents proteasome inhibitor–induced mitochondrial dysfunction and cell death, but protection is lost with mutations found in Parkinson's disease patients[129]. These observations raise the possibility that mutations in PINK1 could render neurons vulnerable to agents, such as abnormal proteins and toxins, that act on proteasomes to induce cell death. PINK1 mutations could also impair mitochondrial function and diminish ATP production necessary for normal UPS function. It is interesting that familial Parkinson's disease–related mutations in PINK1 have been found in normal control subjects who do not have clinical features of parkinsonism[131], again raising the possibility that multiple factors may be necessary for the development of Parkinson's disease .

LRRK2/DARDARIN

In 2002, a large Japanese family with autosomal-dominant Parkinson's disease (incomplete penetrance) was linked to a mutation on chromosome 12p11.2-q13.1 (PARK8)[132]. This mutation was subsequently confirmed in other families[51–58,133]. Recently, two papers reported that Parkinson's disease in these patients was associated with missense mutations in the gene that encodes for the protein leucine-rich repeat kinase 2 (LRRK2), also known as dardarin (from the Basque word for tremor)[134,135]. Not all subjects with these mutations developed Parkinson's disease, suggesting the possible requirement of other contributing etiological factors[136].

Patients with dardarin/LRRK2 mutations have a clinical phenotype similar to sporadic Parkinson's disease with an age of onset ranging from 35–78 years, older than has been described with other gene mutations associated with Parkinson's disease. It has been estimated that the LRRK2 mutation might account for as many as 7% of familial cases and 1.5–3% of cases of apparent sporadic Parkinson's disease[130,133,134]. The pathology of LRRK2-linked familial Parkinson's disease is highly variable. All subjects show nigrostriatal degeneration, but some have Lewy bodies in the SNc while others do not; some have extensive cortical Lewy bodies consistent with a diagnosis of DLB; and some have tau-immunoreactive glial and neuronal inclusions[132,135,137].

LRRK2 is widely expressed throughout the brain[134], but its normal function is not known. LRRK2 resembles the family of tyrosine-like kinases and is predicted to encode a 2482/2527-amino-acid protein that, based on sequence homology with other proteins, appears to be a cytoplasmic kinase[134,135].

It is not known how mutations in DJ-1 cause cell death, however, predictions based on its sequence suggest that the mutation might lead to increased kinase activity, which could promote altered phosphorylation, misfolding, and aggregation of protein substrates. Indeed, recent *in vitro* kinase assays using full-length, recombinant LRRK2 reveal an increase in activity caused by familial-linked mutations in both autophosphorylation and the phosphorylation of a generic substrate. These results suggest a gain-of-function mechanism for LRRK2-linked disease with a central role for kinase activity in the development of Parkinson's disease[138]. Coimmunoprecipitation studies in tissue culture demonstrate that LRRK2 interacts with parkin, but not with α-synuclein; overexpression of wild-type LRRK2 leads to protein aggregates that are increased by coexpression of parkin; and mutant LRRK2 causes neuronal degeneration in both SH-SY5Y cells and primary neuronal cultures[138,139]. It is also noteworthy that some proteins, such as IκB, require phosphorylation as a prerequisite to their ubiquitination and proteasomal degradation[140]. These studies raise the possibility that mutations in LRRK2 lead to altered phosphorylation, changes in UPS function, and increased aggregation of target proteins.

SPORADIC PARKINSON'S DISEASE: ALTERED PROTEASOMAL FUNCTION

There is increasing evidence that proteasomal dysfunction plays a central role in the pathogenesis of Parkinson's disease. This defect might underlie the initiation and/or progression of the neurodegenerative process, and account for other key features of Parkinson's disease, including the occurrence of the various biochemical changes, the formation of Lewy bodies, and the age-related susceptibility of the SNc.

Proteasomal Dysfunction

Parkinson's disease is characterized by protein aggregates and Lewy bodies, so it is reasonable to consider the possibility of protein mishandling and a defect in UPS function. A number of studies have now shown that proteasome structure and function is altered in the SNc in Parkinson's disease. A reduction (approximately 40%) in the content of α-subunits, but not β-subunits, has been found in comparison to age-matched control subjects[141], contrasting with the *increased* expression of α-subunits found in the cerebral cortex (approximately 9%) and striatum (approximately 29%). Immunohistochemical staining similarly demonstrates reduced expression of 20S proteasomal α-subunits, but not β-subunits, in SNc dopaminergic neurons in Parkinson's disease subjects compared to age-matched controls[141]. While proteasomal enzyme activity resides within the β-subunits of the proteasome, α-subunits are required for normal proteasomal function and, in Parkinson's disease, there is a *reduction* of approximately 45–55% in each of the chymotrypsin-like, trypsin-like, and peptadyl glutamyl peptide hydrolytic (PGPH) proteasomal enzymatic activities as compared to controls[141–144]. In contrast, there is *increased* proteasomal enzyme activity in regions that do not degenerate in Parkinson's disease, such as the frontal cortex, striatum, hippocampus, pons, and cerebellum, suggesting a compensatory response[141–143]. Interestingly, these same findings are observed in mildly affected patients, suggesting that altered proteasomal function occurs early in the pathogenic process in Parkinson's disease[143].

Parkinson's disease is also associated with altered levels of expression of proteasome activators. PA700 is comprised of more than 20 different subunits with varying molecular weights[20]. In the SNc in Parkinson's disease, there was either *no change* (42-, 46-, and 95-kDa bands) or a loss of up to 33% (52.5-, 75-, and 81-kDa bands) in these respective PA700 subunits[141]. In contrast, there was a marked *increase* in the levels of the 81-, 75-, 52.5-, and 42-kDa PA700 subunits in the frontal cortex and/or striatum of Parkinson's disease subjects compared to controls. PA28 expression and immunoreactivity was almost undetectable in the SNc in Parkinson's disease, and significantly less than in controls[141]. Interestingly, levels of the PA28 proteasome activator in control subjects are much lower in the SNc than in other brain regions examined, perhaps contributing to the vulnerability of this region to undergo degeneration in Parkinson's disease[141]. These studies illustrate that proteasomal function is impaired in sporadic Parkinson's disease. They also suggest that there is a compensatory response with up-regulation of proteasomal expression and function in regions that are spared, raising the possibility that affected regions cannot mount a satisfactory compensatory response.

Role of Proteasomal Dysfunction

The relevance of proteasome function to the pathogenesis of Parkinson's disease is supported by *in vitro* and *in vivo* studies showing that administration of proteasome inhibitors induces a selective degeneration of dopamine neurons coupled with the formation of inclusion bodies, which stain positively for both α-synuclein and ubiquitin[54,72,145,146]. More specifically, we have recently shown that systemic administration of the proteasome inhibitors epoxomicin or PSI (Z-Ile-Glu(OtBu)-Ala-Leu-al) induces a model of Parkinson's disease in rats[147]. After a latency of several weeks, animals developed a gradually progressive, levodopa/apomorphine-responsive, Parkinson's disease–like syndrome. Positron emission tomography (PET) demonstrated a progressive loss of dopaminergic nerve terminals in the striatum, and postmortem analyses showed progressive striatal dopamine depletion and neurodegeneration with inclusion bodies in the SNc as well as in the LC, DMN, NBM, and peripheral autonomic neurons. At sites of neurodegeneration, there was a 43–82% inhibition of proteasomal enzyme function, while enzyme activity was up-regulated in areas that did not degenerate, again replicating what is found in Parkinson's disease. Although some laboratories have so far not been able to replicate this finding[148–150], several research groups have also found that systemic exposure of rats and mice to PSI can induce a model of Parkinson's disease[151–156]. This model illustrates that inhibition of proteasomal function closely mirrors the behavioral, imaging, pathologic, and biochemical features of Parkinson's disease and supports the concept that proteasomal dysfunction could be a key factor in the pathogenesis of the disorder.

Cause of Proteasomal Dysfunction

The cause of proteasomal dysfunction in Parkinson's disease is not known. It could result from undiscovered gene mutations or could develop secondary to the other biochemical defects that occur in Parkinson's disease, such as oxidative stress or mitochondrial dysfunction[157–159]. More intriguing is the possibility that proteasomal dysfunction in Parkinson's disease could result from exposure to proteasome inhibitors in the environment[160]. Toxins that inhibit the proteasome can be manufactured by bacteria (e.g., actinomycetes, which infect the below-ground portion of crops)[161,162], fungi (e.g., *Apiospora montagne*, which infests wheat/flour)[163], plants[164–166], and the chemical/pharmaceutical industry[160,167]. Lactacystin and epoxomicin are among the most potent proteasome inhibitors, and are naturally produced by actinomycetes (*Streptomyces*) bacteria, which are found globally in the soil and aquatic habitats of gardens and farmland, and can infect root vegetables (e.g., carrots and potatoes) causing "scab" formation[168,169]. Thus, exposure to proteasome inhibitors could occur through drinking water, contaminated food, or living in a rural environment.

Relationship between the UPS and Other Biochemical Changes in Parkinson's Disease

Defects in UPS function could lead to the development of oxidative stress, mitochondrial damage, inflammation, and apoptosis, such as are found in Parkinson's disease. The UPS play a major role in controlling levels of short-lived regulatory/function proteins that are linked to cellular processes that are affected in Parkinson's disease, including antioxidant defense mechanisms[170,171], mitochondrial activity[172,173], inflammatory responses[174], and antiapoptotic pathways[175]. Indeed, inhibition of proteasomal function has been shown to cause oxidative stress[176], mitochondrial dysfunction[176], proinflammatory reactions[177], and apoptosis[172], and theoretically could account for these findings in Parkinson's disease. Further, cell damage induced by proteasome inhibitors is synergistically increased by oxidative stress or agents that promote protein misfolding [31,157,178–180]. It should also be appreciated that proteasomal damage and UPS dysfunction can occur secondary to oxidative stress and mitochondrial dysfunction, although they might still play an important role in the progressive cycle of events that lead to cell death[175,176,183,186].

Role of Proteasomal Dysfunction in Lewy Body Formation

Lewy bodies are intracytoplasmic inclusions, 8–30 μm in diameter, which are characteristically found at sites of neurodegeneration in Parkinson's disease. In the SNc, the Lewy body has a dense central core surrounded by a light halo when stained with hemotoxylin and eosin. Immunostaining and electron microscopy studies show that the core is comprised of punctate aggregates of ubiquitinated proteins, while the outer region consists of radiating filaments (7–20 nm in diameter) of fibrillar α-synuclein and neurofilaments[29,181]. The mechanism underlying the formation of Lewy bodies and their role in the neurodegenerative process has been the focus of considerable debate. α-Synuclein has been postulated to be fundamental to Lewy body formation, as Lewy bodies are rich in α-synuclein[181,182], and α-synuclein protofibrils promote aggregations and inclusion body formation *in vitro*[92,97]. However, not all protein aggregates or Lewy bodies stain positively for α-synuclein[183] and not all Parkinson's disease cases have Lewy bodies[45,135].

Recent studies suggest that Lewy bodies may form and function in a manner similar to an aggresome. Aggresomes are cytoprotective inclusions that form at the centrosome (a perinuclear structure linked to the microtubular system) in response to excess levels of misfolded proteins[8]. Misfolded and aggregated proteins are transported by way of the microtubular system to the centrosome, which expands to become an aggresome[32,184–187]. Simultaneously, components of the proteasome system are recruited to the aggresome to facilitate the clearance of these unwanted proteins. In Parkinson's disease, it can be hypothesized that the Lewy body is an aggresomal inclusion that cannot adequately clear unwanted proteins because of the impairment in proteasomal function and/or the overwhelming production of mutant/damaged proteins[8,29]. In support of this concept, it is noteworthy that Lewy bodies are structurally similar to aggresomes, stain positively for the centrosome/aggresome-specific markers γ-tubulin and pericentrin, and contain the various UPS components[29]. This concept implies that Lewy body formation is a cytoprotective event aimed at combating proteolytic stress. Indeed, inhibition of inclusion body formation in models of proteolytic stress is associated with more rapid and more severe cell death[188,189]. Failure to ubiquitinate proteins might preclude their transport to the centrosome/aggresome and explain the absence of Lewy bodies in patients with parkin mutations. Lack of this protective response might also account for why parkin patients experience such an early onset of severe neuronal degeneration.

The Role of the Proteasome in the Age-Related Susceptibility of the SNc

There is a propensity to develop proteolytic stress with advancing age, as aging is associated with an increased production of damaged proteins combined with a progressive decline in proteasomal function[190–192]. Specifically, there is an increase in protein carbonyls (oxidatively damaged proteins), and a reduction in 26/20S proteasomal mRNA levels and enzymatic activity[190–194]. Thus, in aging cells, there is increased risk of protein accumulation, aggregation, secondary damage to the proteasomal system, and cell death.

Nerve cells are particularly prone to accumulate abnormal proteins, as they do not regenerate. Among brain cells, the SNc may be most vulnerable to the proteolytic effects of aging because the oxidative metabolism of dopamine promotes free radical formation and protein oxidation[193], proteasomal activity pronouncedly declines[192], and dopamine can interact with α-synuclein to promote the formation of toxic protofibrils and protein aggregation[195,196]. In addition, levels of the PA28 proteasome activator are markedly reduced in the SNc in comparison to other brain regions in normal controls[141]. PA28 is thought to play a particularly important role in the degradation of proteins that have been damaged by oxidative stress. Why dopamine neurons, which are prone to generate a high burden of oxidatively damaged proteins, are deficient in this proteasome activator is puzzling.

Thus, normal aging, particularly in SNc dopamine neurons, is associated with increased formation of damaged proteins and a reduced capacity to degrade them. This suggests that aging SNc neurons are prone to develop proteolytic stress, which may account for their specific vulnerability in Parkinson's disease. Indeed, mild neuronal loss and Lewy bodies are found in the SNc in 10–15% of individuals over the age of 65 years who die without clinical evidence of neurological illness[5,197]. Parkinson's disease may thus represent an extreme in the natural process of age-related proteolytic stress, whereby additional genetic and environmental factors overwhelm the capacity of UPS defense mechanisms to deal with the protein load adequately, and a critical number of neurons degenerate eventually. Studies to assess age-related protein load and proteasomal function in other brain regions that are affected in Parkinson's disease are currently underway.

CONCLUSION

There is increasing genetic, pathologic, and experimental evidence suggesting that the pathogenesis of some familial and sporadic forms of Parkinson's disease may be related to a defect in the capacity of the UPS to clear unwanted proteins, resulting in protein accumulation/aggregation, Lewy body formation, and neuronal death. This hypothesis might also account for some of the biochemical features seen in the Parkinson's disease and the age-related vulnerability of the SNc to degenerate. The concept that failure of the UPS plays a central role in the etiopathogenesis of Parkinson's disease is supported by *in vitro* and *in vivo* laboratory experiments that show that inhibition of UPS function can recapitulate key behavioral, pathological, and biochemical features of Parkinson's disease. The recognition that failure of the UPS to play a central role in the initiation or progression of the pathogenic process in Parkinson's disease raises the possibility that neuroprotective therapies could be developed that target this system. This might be accomplished through drugs or gene therapies aimed at preventing or reversing protein damage/misfolding, or stimulating UPS-mediated protein degradation.

In cells, the synthesis, use, and abuse of proteins inevitably leads to the generation of unwanted proteins. These include short-lived/regulatory, incomplete, mutant, misfolded, denatured, oxidized, and otherwise damaged proteins. Because these products have a high tendency to aggregate, interfere with cellular processes, and induce cytotoxicity, they must be removed to maintain cell viability. The UPS is the primary intracellular mechanism responsible for the degradation and clearance of unwanted proteins[19–22]. This process occurs largely in two sequential steps: ubiquitination/deubiquitination and proteolysis. In the first step, a ubiquitin molecule (a 76-amino-acid/8.5-kDa polypeptide) is attached to the unwanted protein via a covalent isopeptide bond between the carboxy group of the C-terminal residue (Gly) of ubiquitin and an internal Lys residue of the substrate protein. Additional ubiquitin molecules are attached to the previously conjugated ubiquitin (at a Lys residue) in a sequential manner to form a polyubiquitin chain. These reactions require ATP and are mediated by a ubiquitin-activating enzyme (E1), which activates ubiquitin by forming a thioester, a conjugating enzyme (E2) that carries activated ubiquitin as a thioester, and an ubiquitin ligase (E3), which transfers activated ubiquitin to the substrate protein. Selectivity of protein ubiquitination is afforded by the fact that there are many E3 enzymes that are specific for one or only a very few different substrate proteins. Further, some proteins require post-translational modification before they can be ubiquitinated (e.g., phosphorylation of IκB), which provides an additional degree of selectivity. Conjugation of a chain of at least four ubiquitin molecules linked through lysine at 48 (K48) acts as a signal for 26S proteasomal degradation. Monoubiquitination (and polyubiquitination linked through lysine 63, K63) preferentially targets proteins to participate in other cellular functions (e.g., gene expression and transport)[198,199]. Ubiquitinated proteins are recognized by subunits (via the Rpn10/S5a and Rpt5/S6') of the PA700 regulatory cap of the 26S proteasome complex (which is comprised of over 60+ subunits/2.5 MDa)[20,200]. In the second step, polyubiquitinated proteins are deubiquitinated by deubiquitination enzymes (ubiquitin C-terminal hydrolases), unfolded, and translocated into the core of the 26S proteasome complex where they are degraded in an ATP-dependent manner. The degradation products are small peptide fragments (2–25 residues) that undergo hydrolysis by peptidases to produce their constituent amino acids that can then be reused in protein synthesis[23]. Monomeric ubiquitin, which is detached from protein conjugates, is reused in the ubiquitination cycle to facilitate the clearance of other unwanted proteins. Some proteins (e.g., oxidatively damaged proteins and possibly α-synuclein) are degraded directly by the 20S proteasome, the catalytic core of the 26S proteasome, without the need for ubiquitination[24,98–100].

Other processes and components, such as phosphorylation by protein kinases and refolding by HSPs, serve to promote the recognition and degradation of unwanted proteins by the UPS[21,27,28].

Figure 1 shows possible sites where parkin mutations, UCH-L1 mutations, α-synuclein mutations, and proteasomal dysfunction might interfere with normal UPS activity, causing proteolytic stress, protein accumulation, and aggregation, and causing cell death in Parkinson's disease.

REFERENCES

1.   Lang AE, Lozano AM. Parkinson's disease. First of two parts. N Engl J Med. 1998;339:1044-53.

2.   Lang AE, Lozano AM. Parkinson's disease. Second of two parts. N Engl J Med. 1998;339:1130-43.

3.   Marras C, Tanner CT. Epidemiology of Parkinson's disease. In Movement Disorders: Neurologic Principles and Practice. 2nd edition. Edited by Watts RL, Koller WC. New York: McGraw-Hill; 2004:177-95.

4.   Forno LS. Neuropathology of Parkinson's disease. J Neuropathol Exp Neurol. 1996;55:259-72.

5.   Braak H, Del Tredici K, Rub U, de Vos RA, Jansen Steur EN, Braak E. Staging of brain pathology related to sporadic Parkinson's disease. Neurobiol Aging. 2003;24:197-211.

6.   Zarow C, Lyness SA, Mortimer JA, Chui HC. Neuronal loss is greater in the locus coeruleus than nucleus basalis and substantia nigra in Alzheimer and Parkinson diseases. Arch Neurol. 2003;60:337-41.

7.   Wakabayashi K, Takahashi H. Neuropathology of autonomic nervous system in Parkinson's disease. Eur Neurol. 1997;38 Suppl 2:2-7.

8.   Olanow CW, Perl DP, DeMartino GN, McNaught KS. Lewy-body formation is an aggresome-related process: a hypothesis. Lancet Neurol. 2004;3:496-503.

9.   Hattori N, Mizuno Y. Pathogenetic mechanisms of parkin in Parkinson's disease. Lancet. 2004;364:722-4.

10.   Moore DJ, West AB, Dawson VL, Dawson TM. Molecular pathophysiology of Parkinson's disease. Ann Rev Neurosci. 2005;28:57-87.

11.   McNaught KS, Olanow CW. Proteolytic stress: a unifying concept in the etiopathogenesis of familial and sporadic Parkinson's disease. Ann Neurol. 2003;53 Suppl 3:S73-86.

12.   Tanner CM. Is the cause of Parkinson's disease environmental or hereditary? Evidence from twin studies. Adv Neurol. 2003;91:133-42.

13.   Tatton WG, Chalmers-Redman R, Brown D, Tatton N. Apoptosis in Parkinson's disease: signals for neuronal degradation. Ann Neurol. 2003;53 Suppl 3:S61-70; discussion S70-2.

14.   Jenner P. Oxidative stress in Parkinson's disease. Ann Neurol. 2003;53:S26-36; discussion S36-8.

15.   Orth M, Schapira AH. Mitochondrial involvement in Parkinson's disease. Neurochem Int. 2002;40:533-41.

16. McGeer PL, McGeer EG. Inflammation and neurodegeneration in Parkinson's disease. Parkinsonism Relat Disord. 2004;10 Suppl 1:S3-7.

17. Beal MF. Excitotoxicity and nitric oxide in Parkinson's disease pathogenesis. Ann Neurol. 1998;44:S110-4.

18. Petrucelli L, Dawson TM. Mechanism of neurodegenerative disease: role of the ubiquitin proteasome system. Ann Med. 2004;36:315-20.

19. Pickart CM. Mechanisms underlying ubiquitination. Annu Rev Biochem. 2001;70:503-33.

20. Pickart CM, Cohen RE. Proteasomes and their kin: proteases in the machine age. Nat Rev Mol Cell Biol. 2004;5:177-87.

21. Goldberg AL. Protein degradation and protection against misfolded or damaged proteins. Nature. 2003;426:895-9.

22. Ciechanover A. Proteolysis: from the lysosome to ubiquitin and the proteasome. Nat Rev Mol Cell Biol. 2005;6:79-87.

23. Saric T, Graef CI, Goldberg AL. Pathway for degradation of peptides generated by proteasomes: a key role for thimet oligopeptidase and other metallopeptidases. J Biol Chem. 2004;279:46723-32.

24. Grune T, Jung T, Merker K, Davies KJ. Decreased proteolysis caused by protein aggregates, inclusion bodies, plaques, lipofuscin, ceroid, and 'aggresomes' during oxidative stress, aging, and disease. Int J Biochem Cell Biol. 2004;36:2519-30.

25. Holmberg CI, Staniszewski KE, Mensah KN, Matouschek A, Morimoto RI. Inefficient degradation of truncated polyglutamine proteins by the proteasome. EMBO J. 2004;23:4307-18.

26. Venkatraman P, Wetzel R, Tanaka M, Nukina N, Goldberg AL. Eukaryotic proteasomes cannot digest polyglutamine sequences and release them during degradation of polyglutamine-containing proteins. Mol Cell. 2004;14:95-104.

27. Hartl FU, Hayer-Hartl M. Molecular chaperones in the cytosol: from nascent chain to folded protein. Science. 2002;295:1852-8.

28. Muchowski PJ, Wacker JL. Modulation of neurodegeneration by molecular chaperones. Nat Rev Neurosci. 2005;6:11-22.

29. McNaught KS, Shashidharan P, Perl DP, Jenner P, Olanow CW. Aggresome-related biogenesis of Lewy bodies. Eur J Neurosci. 2002;16:2136-48.

30. Rajan RS, Illing ME, Bence NF, Kopito RR. Specificity in intracellular protein aggregation and inclusion body formation. Proc Natl Acad Sci U S A. 2001;98:13060-5.

31. Bence NF, Sampat RM, Kopito RR. Impairment of the ubiquitin-proteasome system by protein aggregation. Science. 2001;292:1552-5.

32. Kopito RR. Aggresomes, inclusion bodies and protein aggregation. Trends Cell Biol. 2000;10:524-30.

33. Bennett EJ, Bence NF, Jayakumar R, Kopito RR. Global impairment of the ubiquitin-proteasome system by nuclear or cytoplasmic protein aggregates precedes inclusion body formation. Mol Cell. 2005;17:351-65.

34. Sherman MY, Goldberg AL. Cellular defenses against unfolded proteins: a cell biologist thinks about neurodegenerative diseases. Neuron 2001;29:15-32.

35. Yamamura Y, Sobue I, Ando K, Iida M, Yanagi T. Paralysis agitans of early onset with marked diurnal fluctuation of symptoms. Neurology. 1973;23:239-44.

36. Matsumine H, et al. Localization of a gene for an autosomal recessive form of juvenile Parkinsonism to chromosome 6q25.2-27. Am J Hum Genet. 1997;60:588-96.

37. Kitada T, et al. Mutations in the parkin gene cause autosomal recessive juvenile parkinsonism. Nature. 1998;392:605-8.

38. Mizuno Y, Hattori N, Mori H, Suzuki T, Tanaka K. Parkin and Parkinson's disease. Curr Opin Neurol. 2001;14:477-82.

39. Shimura H, Hattori N, Kubo S, Mizuno Y, Asakawa S, Minoshima S, Shimizu N, Iwai K, Chiba T, Tanaka K, Suzuki T. Familial Parkinson disease gene product, parkin, is a ubiquitin-protein ligase. Nat Genet. 2000;25:302-5.

40. Shimura, H, Schlossmacher MG, Hattori N, Frosch MP, Trockenbacher A, Schneider R, Mizuno Y, Kosik KS, Selkoe DJ. Ubiquitination of a new form of {alpha}-synuclein by parkin from human brain: implications for Parkinson's disease. Science. 2001;293:263-9.

41. Imai Y, Soda M, Takahashi R. Parkin suppresses unfolded protein stress-induced cell death through its E3 ubiquitin-protein ligase activity. J Biol Chem. 2000;275:35661-4.

42. Imai, Y, Soda M, Inoue H, Hattori N, Mizuno Y, Takahashi R. An unfolded putative transmembrane polypeptide, which can lead to endoplasmic reticulum stress, is a substrate of parkin. Cell. 2001;105:891-902.

43. Zhang Y, et al. Parkin functions as an E2-dependent ubiquitin-protein ligase and promotes the degradation of the synaptic vesicle-associated protein, CDCrel-1. Proc Natl Acad Sci U S A. 2000;97:13354-9.

44. Lucking CB, et al. Association between early-onset Parkinson's disease and mutations in the parkin gene. French Parkinson's Disease Genetics Study Group. N Engl J Med. 2000;342:1560-7.

45. Mori H, Kondo T, Yokochi M, Matsumine H, Nakagawa-Hattori Y, Miyake T, Suda K, Mizuno Y. Pathologic and biochemical studies of juvenile parkinsonism linked to chromosome 6q. Neurology. 1998;51:890-2.

46. Foroud T, Uniacke SK, Liu L, Pankratz N, Rudolph A, Halter C, Shults C, Marder K, Conneally PM, Nichols WC. Heterozygosity for a mutation in the parkin gene leads to later onset Parkinson disease. Neurology. 2003;60:796-801.

47. Farrer M, Chan P, Chen R, Tan L, Lincoln S, Hernandez D, Forno L, Gwinn-Hardy K, Petrucelli L, Hussey J, Singleton A, Tanner C, Hardy J, Langston JW. Lewy bodies and parkinsonism in families with parkin mutations. Ann Neurol. 2001;50:293-300.

48. Horowitz JM, Vernace VA, Myers J, Stachowiak MK, Hanlon DW, Fraley GS, Torres G. Immunodetection of Parkin protein in vertebrate and invertebrate brains: a comparative study using specific antibodies. J Chem Neuroanat. 2001;21:75-93.

49. Sakata E, Yamaguchi Y, Kurimoto E, Kikuchi J, Yokoyama S, Yamada S, Kawahara H, Yokosawa H, Hattori N, Mizuno Y, Tanaka K, Kato K. Parkin binds the Rpn10 subunit of 26S proteasomes through its ubiquitin-like domain. EMBO Rep. 2003;4:301-6.

50. Imai Y, Soda M, Hatakeyama S, Akagi T, Hashikawa T, Nakayama KI, Takahashi R. CHIP is associated with parkin, a gene responsible for familial Parkinson's disease, and enhances its ubiquitin ligase activity. Mol Cell. 2002;10:55-67.

51. Cyr DM, Hohfeld J, Patterson C. Protein quality control: U-box-containing E3 ubiquitin ligases join the fold. Trends Biochem Sci. 2002;27:368-75.

52. Shimura H, et al. Immunohistochemical and subcellular localization of Parkin protein: absence of protein in autosomal recessive juvenile parkinsonism patients. Ann Neurol. 1999;45:668-72.

53. Yang Y, Nishimura I, Imai Y, Takahashi R, Lu B. Parkin suppresses dopaminergic neuron-selective neurotoxicity induced by Pael-R in Drosophila. Neuron. 2003;37:911-24.

54. Petrucelli L, O'Farrell C, Lockhart PJ, Baptista M, Kehoe K, Vink L, Choi P, Wolozin B, Farrer M, Hardy J, Cookson MR. Parkin protects against the toxicity associated with mutant alpha-synuclein: proteasome dysfunction selectively affects catecholaminergic neurons. Neuron. 2002;36:1007-19.

55. Itier JM, Ibanez P, Mena MA, Abbas N, Cohen-Salmon C, Bohme GA, Laville M, Pratt J, Corti O, Pradier L, Ret G, Joubert C, Periquet M, Araujo F, Negroni J, Casarejos MJ, Canals S, Solano R, Serrano A, Gallego E, Sanchez M, Denefle P, Benavides J, Tremp G, Rooney TA, Brice A, Garcia de Yebenes J. Parkin gene inactivation alters behaviour and dopamine neurotransmission in the mouse. Hum Mol Genet. 2003;12:2277-91.

56. Goldberg MS, Fleming SM, Palacino JJ, Cepeda C, Lam HA, Bhatnagar A, Meloni EG, Wu N, Ackerson LC, Klapstein GJ, Gajendiran M, Roth BL, Chesselet MF, Maidment NT, Levine MS, Shen J. Parkin-deficient mice exhibit nigrostriatal deficits but not loss of dopaminergic neurons. J Biol Chem. 2003;278:43628-35.

57. Von Coelln R, Thomas B, Savitt JM, Lim KL, Sasaki M, Hess EJ, Dawson VL, Dawson TM. Loss of locus coeruleus neurons and reduced startle in parkin null mice. Proc Natl Acad Sci U S A. 2004;101:10744-9.

58. Perez FA, Palmiter RD. Parkin-deficient mice are not a robust model of parkinsonism. Proc Natl Acad Sci U S A. 2005;102:2174-9.

59. Pesah Y, Pham T, Burgess H, Middlebrooks B, Verstreken P, Zhou Y, Harding M, Bellen H, Mardon G. Drosophila parkin mutants have decreased mass and cell size and increased sensitivity to oxygen radical stress. Development. 2004;131:2183-94.

60. Lincoln SJ, Maraganore DM, Lesnick TG, Bounds R, de Andrade M, Bower JH, Hardy JA, Farrer MJ. Parkin variants in North American Parkinson's disease: cases and controls. Mov Disord. 2003;18:1306-11.

61. Leroy E, Boyer R, Auburger G, Leube B, Ulm G, Mezey E, Harta G, Brownstein MJ, Jonnalagada S, Chernova T, Dehejia A, Lavedan C, Gasser T, Steinbach PJ, Wilkinson KD, Polymeropoulos MH. The ubiquitin pathway in Parkinson's disease. Nature. 1998;395:451-2.

62. Auberger, P. Is the PARK5 I93M mutation a cause of Parkinson's disease with cognitive deficits and cortical Lewy pathology? 16th International Congress on Parkinsonism and Related Disorders Berlin, PT042; 2005.

63. Wintermeyer P, Kruger R, Kuhn W, Muller T, Woitalla D, Berg D, Becker G, Leroy E, Polymeropoulos M, Berger K, Przuntek H, Schols L, Epplen JT, Riess O. Mutation analysis and association studies of the UCHL1 gene in German Parkinson's disease patients. Neuroreport. 2000;11:2079-82.

64. Maraganore DM, Lesnick TG, Elbaz A, Chartier-Harlin MC, Gasser T, Kruger R, Hattori N, Mellick GD, Quattrone A, Satoh J, Toda T, Wang

J, Ioannidis JP, de Andrade M, Rocca WA. UCHL1 is a Parkinson's disease susceptibility gene. Ann Neuron. 2004;55:512-21.

65. Healy DG, Abou-Sleiman PM, Casas JP, Ahmadi KR, Lynch T, Gandhi S, Muqit MM, Foltynie T, Barker R, Bhatia KP, Quinn NP, Lees AJ, Gibson JM, Holton JL, Revesz T, Goldstein DB, Wood NW. UCHL-1 is not a Parkinson's disease susceptibility gene. Ann Neurol. 2006;59:627-33.

66. Solano SM, Miller DW, Augood SJ, Young AB, Penney JB Jr. Expression of alpha-synuclein, parkin, and ubiquitin carboxy-terminal hydrolase L1 mRNA in human brain: genes associated with familial Parkinson's disease. Ann Neurol. 2000;47:201-10.

67. Wilkinson KD, Deshpande S, Larsen CN. Comparisons of neuronal (PGP 9.5) and non-neuronal ubiquitin C-terminal hydrolases. Biochem Soc Trans. 1992;20:631-7.

68. Wilkinson KD, Lee KM, Deshpande S, Duerksen-Hughes P, Boss JM, Pohl J. The neuron-specific protein PGP 9.5 is a ubiquitin carboxyl-terminal hydrolase. Science. 1989;246:670-3.

69. Liu Y, Fallon L, Lashuel HA, Liu Z, Lansbury PT Jr. The UCH-L1 gene encodes two opposing enzymatic activities that affect alpha-synuclein degradation and Parkinson's disease susceptibility. Cell. 2002;111:209-18.

70. Nishikawa K, Li H, Kawamura R, Osaka H, Wang YL, Hara Y, Hirokawa T, Manago Y, Amano T, Noda M, Aoki S, Wada K. Alterations of structure and hydrolase activity of parkinsonism-associated human ubiquitin carboxyl-terminal hydrolase L1 variants. Biochem Biophys Res Commun. 2003;304:176-83.

71. Osaka, H, Wang YL, Takada K, Takizawa S, Setsuie R, Li H, Sato Y, Nishikawa K, Sun YJ, Sakurai M, Harada T, Hara Y, Kimura I, Chiba S, Namikawa K, Kiyama H, Noda M, Aoki S, Wada K. Ubiquitin carboxy-terminal hydrolase L1 binds to and stabilizes monoubiquitin in neuron. Hum Mol Genet. 2003;12:1945-58.

72. McNaught KS, Mytilineou C, Jnobaptiste R, Yabut J, Shashidharan P, Jennert P, Olanow CW. Impairment of the ubiquitin-proteasome system causes dopaminergic cell death and inclusion body formation in ventral mesencephalic cultures. J Neurochem. 2002;81:301-6.

73. Saigoh K, Wang YL, Suh JG, Yamanishi T, Sakai Y, Kiyosawa H, Harada T, Ichihara N, Wakana S, Kikuchi T, Wada K. Intragenic deletion in the gene encoding ubiquitin carboxy-terminal hydrolase in gad mice. Nat Genet. 1999;23:47-51.

74. Golbe LI, Di Iorio G, Bonavita V, Miller DC, Duvoisin RC. A large kindred with autosomal dominant Parkinson's disease. Ann Neurol. 1990;27:276-82.

75. Polymeropoulos MH, Higgins JJ, Golbe LI, Johnson WG, Ide SE, Di Iorio G, Sanges G, Stenroos ES, Pho LT, Schaffer AA, Lazzarini AM, Nussbaum RL, Duvoisin RC. Mapping of a gene for Parkinson's disease to chromosome 4q21-q23. Science. 1996;274:1197-9.

76. Polymeropoulos MH, Lavedan C, Leroy E, Ide SE, Dehejia A, Dutra A, Pike B, Root H, Rubenstein J, Boyer R, Stenroos ES, Chandrasekharappa S, Athanassiadou A, Papapetropoulos T, Johnson WG, Lazzarini AM, Duvoisin RC, Di Iorio G, Golbe LI, Nussbaum RL. Mutation in the alpha-synuclein gene identified in families with Parkinson's disease. Science. 1997;276:2045-7.

77. Kruger R, Kuhn W, Muller T, Woitalla D, Graeber M, Kosel S, Przuntek H, Epplen JT, Schols L, Riess O. Ala30Pro mutation in the gene encoding alpha-synuclein in Parkinson's disease. Nat Genet. 1998;18:106-8.

78. Zarranz JJ, Alegre J, Gomez-Esteban JC, Lezcano E, Ros R, Ampuero I, Vidal L, Hoenicka J, Rodriguez O, Atares B, Llorens V, Gomez Tortosa E, del Ser T, Munoz DG, de Yebenes JG. The new mutation, E46K, of alpha-synuclein causes Parkinson and Lewy body dementia. Ann Neurol. 2004;55:164-73.

79. Chartier-Harlin MC, Kachergus J, Roumier C, Mouroux V, Douay X, Lincoln S, Levecque C, Larvor L, Andrieux J, Hulihan M, Waucquier N, Defebvre L, Amouyel P, Farrer M, Destee A. Alpha-synuclein locus duplication as a cause of familial Parkinson's disease. Lancet. 2004;364:1167-9.

80. Ibanez P, Bonnet AM, Debarges B, Lohmann E, Tison F, Pollak P, Agid Y, Durr A, Brice A. Causal relation between alpha-synuclein gene duplication and familial Parkinson's disease. Lancet. 2004;364:1169-71.

81. Singleton AB, Farrer M, Johnson J, Singleton A, Hague S, Kachergus J, Hulihan M, Peuralinna T, Dutra A, Nussbaum R, Lincoln S, Crawley A, Hanson M, Maraganore D, Adler C, Cookson MR, Muenter M, Baptista M, Miller D, Blancato J, Hardy J, Gwinn-Hardy K. alpha-Synuclein locus triplication causes Parkinson's disease. Science. 2003;302:841.

82. Muenter MD, Forno LS, Hornykiewicz O, Kish SJ, Maraganore DM, Caselli RJ, Okazaki H, Howard FM Jr, Snow BJ, Calne DB. Hereditary form of parkinsonism--dementia. Ann Neurol. 1998;43:768-81.

83. Miller DW, Hague SM, Clarimon J, Baptista M, Gwinn-Hardy K, Cookson MR, Singleton AB. Alpha-synuclein in blood and brain from familial Parkinson disease with SNCA locus triplication. Neurology. 2004;62:1835-8.

84. Farrer M, Kachergus J, Forno L, Lincoln S, Wang DS, Hulihan M, Maraganore D, Gwinn-Hardy K, Wszolek Z, Dickson D, Langston JW. Comparison of kindreds with parkinsonism and alpha-synuclein genomic multiplications. Ann Neurol. 2004;55:174-9.

85. Kotzbauer PT, Giasson BI, Kravitz AV, Golbe LI, Mark MH, Trojanowski JQ, Lee VM. Fibrillization of alpha-synuclein and tau in familial Parkinson's disease caused by the A53T alpha-synuclein mutation. Exp Neurol. 2004;187:279-88.

86. Duda JE, Giasson BI, Mabon ME, Miller DC, Golbe LI, Lee VM, Trojanowski JQ. Concurrence of alpha-synuclein and tau brain pathology in the Contursi kindred. Acta Neuropathol (Berl). 2002;104:7-11.

87. Maroteaux L, Campanelli JT, Scheller RH. Synuclein: a neuron-specific protein localized to the nucleus and presynaptic nerve terminal. J Neurosci. 1988;8:2804-15.

88. Jakes R, Spillantini MG, Goedert M. Identification of two distinct synucleins from human brain. FEBS Lett. 1994;345:27-32.

89. Goedert M. Alpha-synuclein and neurodegenerative diseases. Nat Rev Neurosci. 2001;2:492-501.

90. Abeliovich A, Schmitz Y, Farinas I, Choi-Lundberg D, Ho WH, Castillo PE, Shinsky N, Verdugo JM, Armanini M, Ryan A, Hynes M, Phillips H, Sulzer D, Rosenthal A. Mice lacking alpha-synuclein display functional deficits in the nigrostriatal dopamine system. Neuron. 2000;25:239-52.

91. Chandra S, Fornai F, Kwon HB, Yazdani U, Atasoy D, Liu X, Hammer RE, Battaglia G, German DC, Castillo PE, Sudhof TC. Double-knockout mice for alpha- and beta-synucleins: effect on synaptic functions. Proc Natl Acad Sci U S A. 2004;101:14966-71.

92. Conway KA, Harper JD, Lansbury PT. Accelerated in vitro fibril formation by a mutant alpha-synuclein linked to early-onset Parkinson disease. Nat Med. 1998;4:1318-20.

93. Weinreb PH, Zhen W, Poon AW, Conway KA, Lansbury PT Jr. NACP, a protein implicated in Alzheimer's disease and learning, is natively unfolded. Biochemistry. 1996;35:13709-15.

94. Conway KA, Lee SJ, Rochet JC, Ding TT, Williamson RE, Lansbury PT Jr. Acceleration of oligomerization, not fibrillization, is a shared property of both alpha-synuclein mutations linked to early-onset

Parkinson's disease: implications for pathogenesis and therapy. Proc Natl Acad Sci U S A. 2000;97:571-6.

95. Li J, Uversky VN, Fink AL. Effect of familial Parkinson's disease point mutations A30P and A53T on the structural properties, aggregation, and fibrillation of human alpha-synuclein. Biochemistry. 2001;40:11604-13.

96. Lashuel HA, Petre BM, Wall J, Simon M, Nowak RJ, Walz T, Lansbury PT Jr. Alpha-synuclein, especially the Parkinson's disease-associated mutants, forms pore-like annular and tubular protofibrils. J Mol Biol. 2002;322:1089-102.

97. Caughey B, Lansbury PT. Protofibrils, pores, fibrils, and neurodegeneration: separating the responsible protein aggregates from the innocent bystanders. Annu Rev Neurosci. 2003;26:267-98.

98. Bennett MC, Bishop JF, Leng Y, Chock PB, Chase TN, Mouradian MM. Degradation of alpha-synuclein by proteasome. J Biol Chem. 1999;274:33855-8.

99. Tofaris GK, Layfield R, Spillantini MG. alpha-Synuclein metabolism and aggregation is linged to ubiqutin-independent degradation by the proteasome. FEBS Lett. 2001; 509:22-6

100. Liu CW, Corboy MJ, DeMartino GN, Thomas PJ. Endoproteolytic activity of the proteasome. Science. 2003;299:408-11.

101. Tanaka Y, Engelender S, Igarashi S, Rao RK, Wanner T, Tanzi RE, Sawa A, L Dawson V, Dawson TM, Ross CA. Inducible expression of mutant alpha-synuclein decreases proteasome activity and increases sensitivity to mitochondria-dependent apoptosis. Hum Mol Genet. 2001;10:919-26.

102. Stefanis L, Larsen KE, Rideout HJ, Sulzer D, Greene LA. Expression of A53T mutant but not wild-type alpha-synuclein in PC12 cells induces alterations of the ubiquitin-dependent degradation system, loss of dopamine release, and autophagic cell death. J Neurosci. 2001;21:9549-60.

103. Snyder H, Mensah K, Theisler C, Lee J, Matouschek A, Wolozin B. Aggregated and monomeric alpha-synuclein bind to the S6' proteasomal protein and inhibit proteasomal function. J Biol Chem. 2003;278:11753-9.

104. Liu CW, Giasson BI, Lewis KA, Lee VM, Demartino GN, Thomas PJ. A precipitating role for truncated alpha-synuclein and the proteasome in alpha-synuclein aggregation: implications for pathogenesis of Parkinson's disease. J Biol Chem. 2005;280(24):22670-8.

105. Fernagut PO, Chesselet MF. Alpha-synuclein and transgenic mouse models. Neurobiol Dis. 2004;17:123-30.

106. Lee M, Hyun D, Halliwell B, Jenner P. Effect of the overexpression of wild-type or mutant alpha-synuclein on cell susceptibility to insult. J Neurochem. 2001;76:998-1009.

107. Feany MB, Bender WW. A Drosophila model of Parkinson's disease. Nature. 2000;404:394-8.

108. Kirik D, Annett LE, Burger C, Muzyczka N, Mandel RJ, Bjorklund A. Nigrostriatal alpha-synucleinopathy induced by viral vector-mediated overexpression of human alpha-synuclein: a new primate model of Parkinson's disease. Proc Natl Acad Sci U S A. 2003;100:2884-9.

109. Lee HJ, Khoshaghideh F, Patel S, Lee SJ. Clearance of alpha-synuclein oligomeric intermediates via the lysosomal degradation pathway. J Neurosci. 2004;24:1888-96.

110. Cuervo AM, Stefanis L, Fredenburg R, Lansbury PT, Sulzer D. Impaired degradation of mutant alpha-synuclein by chaperone-mediated autophagy. Science. 2004;305:1292-5.

111. van Duijn CM, Dekker MC, Bonifati V, Galjaard RJ, Houwing-Duistermaat JJ, Snijders PJ, Testers L, Breedveld GJ, Horstink M, Sandkuijl LA, van Swieten JC, Oostra BA, Heutink P. Park7, a novel locus for autosomal recessive early-onset parkinsonism, on chromosome 1p36. Am J Hum Genet. 2001;69:629-34.

112. Bonifati V, Rizzu P, van Baren MJ, Schaap O, Breedveld GJ, Krieger E, Dekker MC, Squitieri F, Ibanez P, Joosse M, van Dongen JW, Vanacore N, van Swieten JC, Brice A, Meco G, van Duijn CM, Oostra BA, Heutink P. Mutations in the DJ-1 gene associated with autosomal recessive early-onset parkinsonism. Science. 2003;299:256-9.

113. Bonifati V, Oostra BA, Heutink P. Linking DJ-1 to neurodegeneration offers novel insights for understanding the pathogenesis of Parkinson's disease. J Mol Med. 2004;82:163-74.

114. Nagakubo D, Taira T, Kitaura H, Ikeda M, Tamai K, Iguchi-Ariga SM, Ariga H. DJ-1, a novel oncogene which transforms mouse NIH3T3 cells in cooperation with ras. Biochem Biophys Res Commun. 1997;231:509-13.

115. Abou-Sleiman PM, Healy DG, Quinn N, Lees AJ, Wood, NW. The role of pathogenic DJ-1 mutations in Parkinson's disease. Ann Neurol. 2003;54:283-6.

116. Shang H, Lang D, Jean-Marc B, Kaelin-Lang A. Localization of DJ-1 mRNA in the mouse brain. Neurosci Lett. 2004;367:273-7.

117. Bandopadhyay R, Kingsbury AE, Cookson MR, Reid AR, Evans IM, Hope AD, Pittman AM, Lashley T, Canet-Aviles R, Miller DW, McLendon C, Strand C, Leonard AJ, Abou-Sleiman PM, Healy DG, Ariga H, Wood NW, de Silva R, Revesz T, Hardy JA, Lees AJ. The expression of DJ-1 (PARK7) in normal human CNS and idiopathic Parkinson's disease. Brain. 2004;127:420-30.

118. Yokota T, Sugawara K, Ito K, Takahashi R, Ariga H, Mizusawa H. Down regulation of DJ-1 enhances cell death by oxidative stress, ER stress, and proteasome inhibition. Biochem Biophys Res Commun. 2003;312:1342-8.

119. Taira T, Saito Y, Niki T, Iguchi-Ariga SM, Takahashi K, Ariga H. DJ-1 has a role in antioxidative stress to prevent cell death. EMBO Rep. 2004;5:213-8.

120. Olzmann JA, Brown K, Wilkinson KD, Rees HD, Huai Q, Ke H, Levey AI, Li L, Chin LS. Familial Parkinson's disease-associated L166P mutation disrupts DJ-1 protein folding and function. J Biol Chem. 2004;279:8506-15.

121. Lee SJ, Kim SJ, Kim IK, Ko J, Jeong CS, Kim GH, Park C, Kang SO, Suh PG, Lee HS, Cha SS. Crystal structures of human DJ-1 and Escherichia coli Hsp31, which share an evolutionarily conserved domain. J Biol Chem. 2003;278:44552-9.

122. Wilson MA, St Amour CV, Collins JL, Ringe D, Petsko GA. The 1.8-A resolution crystal structure of YDR533Cp from Saccharomyces cerevisiae: a member of the DJ-1/ThiJ/PfpI superfamily. Proc Natl Acad Sci U S A. 2004;101:1531-6.

123. Moore DJ, et al. Association of DJ-1 and parkin mediated by pathogenic DJ-1 mutations and oxidative stress. Hum Mol Genet. 2005;14:71-84.

124. Moore DJ, Zhang L, Dawson TM, Dawson VL. A missense mutation (L166P) in DJ-1, linked to familial Parkinson's disease, confers reduced protein stability and impairs homo-oligomerization. J Neurochem. 2003;87:1558-67.

125. Shendelman S, Jonason A, Martinat C, Leete T, Abeliovich A. DJ-1 is a redox-dependent molecular chaperone that inhibits alpha-synuclein aggregate formation. PLoS Biol. 2004;2:e362.

126. Goldberg MS, Pisani A, Haburcak M, Vortherms TA, Kitada T, Costa C, Tong Y, Martella G, Tscherter A, Martins A, Bernardi G, Roth BL, Pothos EN, Calabresi P, Shen J. Nigrostriatal dopaminergic deficits and hypokinesia caused by inactivation of the familial parkinsonism-linked gene DJ-1. Neuron. 2005;45:489-96.

127. Valente EM, Bentivoglio AR, Dixon PH, Ferraris A, Ialongo T, Frontali M, Albanese A, Wood NW. Localization of a novel locus for autosomal recessive early-onset parkinsonism, PARK6, on human chromosome 1p35-p36. Am J Hum Genet. 2001;68:895-900.

128. Valente EM, Brancati F, Ferraris A, Graham EA, Davis MB, Breteler MM, Gasser T, Bonifati V, Bentivoglio AR, De Michele G, Durr A, Cortelli P, Wassilowsky D, Harhangi BS, Rawal N, Caputo V, Filla A, Meco G, Oostra BA, Brice A, Albanese A, Dallapiccola B, Wood NW. PARK6-linked parkinsonism occurs in several European families. Ann Neurol. 2002;51:14-8.

129. Valente EM, Abou-Sleiman PM, Caputo V, Muqit MM, Harvey K, Gispert S, Ali Z, Del Turco D, Bentivoglio AR, Healy DG, Albanese A, Nussbaum R, Gonzalez-Maldonado R, Deller T, Salvi S, Cortelli P, Gilks WP, Latchman DS, Harvey RJ, Dallapiccola B, Auburger G, Wood NW. Hereditary early-onset Parkinson's disease caused by mutations in PINK1. Science. 2004;304:1158-60.

130. Healy DG, Abou-Sleiman PM, Wood NW. PINK, PANK, or PARK? A clinicians' guide to familial parkinsonism. Lancet Neurol. 2004;3:652-62.

131. Rogaeva E, Johnson J, Lang AE, Gulick C, Gwinn-Hardy K, Kawarai T, Sato C, Morgan A, Werner J, Nussbaum R, Petit A, Okun MS, McInerney A, Mandel R, Groen JL, Fernandez HH, Postuma R, Foote KD, Salehi-Rad S, Liang Y, Reimsnider S, Tandon A, Hardy J, St George-Hyslop P, Singleton AB. Analysis of the PINK1 gene in a large cohort of cases with Parkinson disease. Arch Neurol. 2004;61:1898-904.

132. Funayama M, Hasegawa K, Kowa H, Saito M, Tsuji S, Obata F. A new locus for Parkinson's disease (PARK8) maps to chromosome 12p11.2-q13.1. Ann Neurol. 2002;51:296-301.

133. Nichols WC, Pankratz N, Hernandez D, Paisan-Ruiz C, Jain S, Halter CA, Michaels VE, Reed T, Rudolph A, Shults CW, Singleton A, Foroud T. Genetic screening for a single common LRRK2 mutation in familial Parkinson's disease. Lancet. 2005;365:410-2.

134. Paisan-Ruiz C, Jain S, Evans EW, Gilks WP, Simon J, van der Brug M, Lopez de Munain A, Aparicio S, Gil AM, Khan N, Johnson J, Martinez JR, Nicholl D, Carrera IM, Pena AS, de Silva R, Lees A, Marti-Masso JF, Perez-Tur J, Wood NW, Singleton AB. Cloning of the gene containing mutations that cause PARK8-linked Parkinson's disease. Neuron 2004;44:595-600.

135. Zimprich A, Biskup S, Leitner P, Lichtner P, Farrer M, Lincoln S, Kachergus J, Hulihan M, Uitti RJ, Calne DB, Stoessl AJ, Pfeiffer RF,

Patenge N, Carbajal IC, Vieregge P, Asmus F, Muller-Myhsok B, Dickson DW, Meitinger T, Strom TM, Wszolek ZK, Gasser T. Mutations in LRRK2 cause autosomal-dominant parkinsonism with pleomorphic pathology. Neuron. 2004;44:601-7.

136. Di Fonzo A, Rohe CF, Ferreira J, Chien HF, Vacca L, Stocchi F, Guedes L, Fabrizio E, Manfredi M, Vanacore N, Goldwurm S, Breedveld G, Sampaio C, Meco G, Barbosa E, Oostra BA, Bonifati V. A frequent LRRK2 gene mutation associated with autosomal dominant Parkinson's disease. Lancet. 2005;365:412-5.

137. Wszolek ZK, Pfeiffer RF, Tsuboi Y, Uitti RJ, McComb RD, Stoessl AJ, Strongosky AJ, Zimprich A, Muller-Myhsok B, Farrer MJ, Gasser T, Calne DB, Dickson DW Autosomal dominant parkinsonism associated with variable synuclein and tau pathology. Neurology. 2004;62:1619-22.

138. Smith WW, Pei Z, Jiang H, Moore DJ, Liang Y, West AB, Dawson VL, Dawson TM, Ross CA. Leucine-rich repeat kinase 2 (LRRK2) interacts with parkin, and mutant LRRK2 induces neuronal degeneration. Proc Natl Acad Sci U S A. 2005;102:18676-81.

139. West AB, Moore DJ, Biskup S, Bugayenko A, Smith WW, Ross CA, Dawson VL, Dawson TM. Parkinson's disease-associated mutations in leucine-rich repeat kinase 2 augment kinase activity. Proc Natl Acad Sci U S A. 2005;102:16842-7.

140. DiDonato J, Mercurio F, Rosette C, Wu-Li J, Suyang H, Ghosh S, Karin M. Mapping of the inducible IkappaB phosphorylation sites that signal its ubiquitination and degradation. Mol Cell Biol. 1996;16:1295-304.

141. McNaught KS, Belizaire R, Isacson O, Jenner P, Olanow CW. Altered proteasomal function in sporadic Parkinson's disease. Exp Neurol. 2003;179:38-46.

142. McNaught KS, Jenner P. Proteasomal function is impaired in substantia nigra in Parkinson's disease. Neurosci Lett. 2001;297:191-4.

143. Tofaris GK, Razzaq A, Ghetti B, Lilley K, Spillantini MG. Ubiquitination of alpha-synuclein in Lewy bodies is a pathological event not associated with impairment of proteasome function. J Biol Chem. 2003;278:44405-11.

144. Furukawa Y, Vigouroux S, Wong H, Guttman M, Rajput AH, Ang L, Briand M, Kish SJ, Briand Y. Brain proteasomal function in sporadic Parkinson's disease and related disorders. Ann Neurol. 2002;51:779-82.

145. McNaught KSP, Bjorklund LM, Belizaire R, Jenner P, Olanow CW. Proteasome inhibition causes nigral degeneration with inclusion bodies in rats. NeuroReport. 2002;13:1437-41.

146. Fornai F, Lenzi P, Gesi M, Ferrucci M, Lazzeri G, Busceti CL, Ruffoli R, Soldani P, Ruggieri S, Alessandri MG, Paparelli A. Fine structure and biochemical mechanisms underlying nigrostriatal inclusions and cell death after proteasome inhibition. J Neurosci. 2003;23:8955-66.

147. McNaught KSP, Perl DP, Brownell AL, Olanow CW. Systemic exposure to proteasome inhibitors causes a progressive model of Parkinson's disease. Ann Neurol. 2004;56:149-62.

148. Kordower JH, Kanaan NM, Chu Y, Suresh Babu R, Stansell J 3rd, Terpstra BT, Sortwell CE, Steece-Collier K, Collier TJ. Failure of proteasome inhibitor administration to provide a model of Parkinson's disease in rats and monkeys. Ann Neurol. 2006;60:264-8.

149. Bove J, Zhou C, Jackson-Lewis V, Taylor J, Chu Y, Rideout HJ, Wu DC, Kordower JH, Petrucelli L, Przedborski S. Proteasome inhibition and Parkinson's disease modeling. Ann Neurol. 2006;60:260-4.

150. Manning-Bog AB, Reaney SH, Chou VP, Johnston LC, McCormack AL, Johnston J, Langston JW, Di Monte DA. Lack of nigrostriatal pathology in a rat model of proteasome inhibition. Ann Neurol. 2006;60:256-60.

151. Zeng BY, Bukhatwa S, Hikima A, Rose S, Jenner P. Reproducible nigral cell loss after systemic proteasomal inhibitor administration to rats. Ann Neurol 2006;60:248-52.

152. Schapira AH, Cleeter MW, Muddle JR, Workman JM, Cooper JM, King RH. Proteasomal inhibition causes loss of nigral tyrosine hydroxylase neurons. Ann Neurol. 2006;60:253-5.

153. Miwa H, Kubo T, Suzuki A, Kondo T. Intragastric proteasome inhibition induces alpha-synuclein-immunopositive aggregations in neurons in the dorsal motor nucleus of the vagus in rats. Neurosci Lett. 2006;401:146-9.

154. Thomas A, McNaught KS, Gonzalez-Maeso J, Sealfon SC, Olanow CW. PSI induces proteasome inhibition and motor disturbances in rats. Mov Disord. 2006;21 Suppl:P80.

155. Nair VD, McNaught KS, Gonzalez-Maeso J, Sealfon SC, Olanow CW. p53 Mediates non-transcriptional cell death in dopaminergic cells in response to proteasome inhibition. J Biol Chem. 281(51):39550-60.

156. Crotty S. Treatment with a novel phospholipid-based drug formulation prevents behavioral deficits induced by proteasome inhibition: implication for Parkinson's disease. Soc Neurosci. 379/MM91; 2006.

157. Bulteau AL. Oxidative modification and inactivation of the proteasome during coronary occlusion/reperfusion. J Biol Chem. 2001;276:30057-63.

158. Hendil KB, Hartmann-Petersen R, Tanaka K. 26S proteasomes function as stable entities. J Mol Biol. 2002;315:627-36.

159. Jenner P, Olanow CW. Understanding cell death in Parkinson's disease. Ann Neurol. 1998;44:S72-84.

160. Kisselev AF, Goldberg AL. Proteasome inhibitors: from research tools to drug candidates. Chem Biol. 2001;8:739-58.

161. Fenteany G, Schreiber SL. Lactacystin, proteasome function, and cell fate. J Biol Chem. 1998;273:8545-8.

162. Sin N, Kim KB, Elofsson M, Meng L, Auth H, Kwok BH, Crews CM. Total synthesis of the potent proteasome inhibitor epoxomicin: a useful tool for understanding proteasome biology. Bioorg Med Chem Lett. 1999;9:2283-8.

163. Koguchi Y, Kohno J, Nishio M, Takahashi K, Okuda T, Ohnuki T, Komatsubara S. TMC-95A, B, C, and D, novel proteasome inhibitors produced by Apiospora montagnei Sacc. TC 1093. Taxonomy, production, isolation, and biological activities. J Antibiot (Tokyo). 2000;53:105-9.

164. Nam S, Smith DM, Dou QP. Ester bond-containing tea polyphenols potently inhibit proteasome activity in vitro and in vivo. J Biol Chem. 2001;276:13322-30.

165. Kazi A, Urbizu DA, Kuhn DJ, Acebo AL, Jackson ER, Greenfelder GP, Kumar NB, Dou QP. A natural musaceas plant extract inhibits proteasome activity and induces apoptosis selectively in human tumor and transformed, but not normal and non-transformed, cells. Int J Mol Med. 2003;12:879-87.

166. Jana NR, Dikshit P, Goswami A, Nukina, N. Inhibition of proteasomal function by curcumin induces apoptosis through mitochondrial pathway. J Biol Chem. 2004;279:11680-5.

167. Zhou Y, Shie FS, Piccardo P, Montine TJ, Zhang J. Proteasomal inhibition induced by manganese ethylene-bis-dithiocarbamate: relevance to Parkinson's disease. Neuroscience. 2004;128:281-91.

168. Ensign JC, Normand P, Burden JP, Yallop CA. Physiology of some actinomycete genera. Res Microbiol. 1993;144:657-60.

169. Cross T. Aquatic actinomycetes: a critical survey of the occurrence, growth and role of actinomycetes in aquatic habitats. J Appl Bacteriol. 1981;50:397-423.

170. Atlante A, Bobba A, Calissano P, Passarella S, Marra E. The apoptosis/necrosis transition in cerebellar granule cells depends on

the mutual relationship of the antioxidant and the proteolytic systems which regulate ROS production and cytochrome c release en route to death. J Neurochem. 2003;84:960-71.

171. Jha N, Kumar MJ, Boonplueang R, Andersen JK. Glutathione decreases in dopaminergic PC12 cells interfere with the ubiquitin protein degradation pathway: relevance for Parkinson's disease? J Neurochem. 2002;80:555-61.

172. Hoglinger GU, Carrard G, Michel PP, Medja F, Lombes A, Ruberg M, Friguet B, Hirsch EC. Dysfunction of mitochondrial complex I and the proteasome: interactions between two biochemical deficits in a cellular model of Parkinson's disease. J Neurochem. 2003;86:1297-307.

173. Lee HJ, Shin SY, Choi C, Lee YH, Lee SJ. Formation and removal of alpha-synuclein aggregates in cells exposed to mitochondrial inhibitors. J Biol Chem. 2002;277(7):5411-7.

174. Li Z, Jansen M, Pierre SR, Figueiredo-Pereira ME. Neurodegeneration: linking ubiquitin/proteasome pathway impairment with inflammation. Int J Biochem Cell Biol. 2003;35:547-52.

175. Jesenberger V, Jentsch S. Deadly encounter: ubiquitin meets apoptosis. Nat Rev Mol Cell Biol. 2002;3:112-21.

176. Kikuchi S, Shinpo K, Tsuji S, Takeuchi M, Yamagishi S, Makita Z, Niino M, Yabe I, Tashiro K. Effect of proteasome inhibitor on cultured mesencephalic dopaminergic neurons. Brain Res. 2003;964:228-36.

177. Rockwell P, Yuan H, Magnusson R, Figueiredo-Pereira ME. Proteasome inhibition in neuronal cells induces a proinflammatory response manifested by upregulation of cyclooxygenase-2, its accumulation as ubiquitin conjugates, and production of the prostaglandin PGE(2). Arch Biochem Biophys. 2000;374:325-33.

178. Sitte N, Merker K, von Zglinicki T, Grune T. Protein oxidation and degradation during proliferative senescence of human MRC-5 fibroblasts. Free Radic Biol Med. 2000;28:701-8.

179. Okada K, Wangpoengtrakul C, Osawa T, Toyokuni S, Tanaka K, Uchida K. 4-Hydroxy-2-nonenal-mediated impairment of intracellular proteolysis during oxidative stress. Identification of proteasomes as target molecules. J Biol Chem. 1999;274:23787-93.

180. Reinheckel T, Sitte N, Ullrich O, Kuckelkorn U, Davies KJ, Grune T. Comparative resistance of the 20S and 26S proteasome to oxidative stress. Biochem J. 1998;335:637-42.

181. Spillantini MG, Crowther RA, Jakes R, Hasegawa M, Goedert M. alpha-Synuclein in filamentous inclusions of Lewy bodies from Parkinson's disease and dementia with lewy bodies. Proc Natl Acad Sci U S A. 1998;95:6469-73.

182. Spillantini MG, Schmidt ML, Lee VM, Trojanowski JQ, Jakes R, Goedert M. Alpha-synuclein in Lewy bodies. Nature. 1997;388:839-40.

183. van Duinen SG, Lammers GJ, Maat-Schieman ML, Roos RA. Numerous and widespread alpha-synuclein-negative Lewy bodies in an asymptomatic patient. Acta Neuropathol (Berl). 1999;97:533-9.

184. Johnston JA, Illing ME, Kopito RR. Cytoplasmic dynein/dynactin mediates the assembly of aggresomes. Cell Motil Cytoskeleton. 2002;53:26-38.

185. Johnston JA, Ward CL, Kopito RR. Aggresomes: a cellular response to misfolded proteins. J Cell Biol. 1998;143:1883-98.

186. Kawaguchi Y, Kovacs JJ, McLaurin A, Vance JM, Ito A, Yao TP. The deacetylase HDAC6 regulates aggresome formation and cell viability in response to misfolded protein stress. Cell. 2003;115:727-38.

187. Arrasate M, Mitra S, Schweitzer ES, Segal MR, Finkbeiner S. Inclusion body formation reduces levels of mutant huntingtin and the risk of neuronal death. Nature. 2004;431:805-10.

188. Taylor JP, Tanaka F, Robitschek J, Sandoval CM, Taye A, Markovic-Plese S, Fischbeck KH. Aggresomes protect cells by enhancing the degradation of toxic polyglutamine-containing protein. Hum Mol Genet. 2003;12:749-57.

189. Cummings CJ, Reinstein E, Sun Y, Antalffy B, Jiang Y, Ciechanover A, Orr HT, Beaudet AL, Zoghbi HY. Mutation of the E6-AP ubiquitin ligase reduces nuclear inclusion frequency while accelerating polyglutamine-induced pathology in SCA1 mice. Neuron. 1999;24:879-92.

190. Keller JN, Dimayuga E, Chen Q, Thorpe J, Gee J, Ding Q. Autophagy, proteasomes, lipofuscin, and oxidative stress in the aging brain. Int J Biochem Cell Biol. 2004;36:2376-91.

191. Keller JN, Hanni KB, Markesbery WR. Possible involvement of proteasome inhibition in aging: implications for oxidative stress. Mech Ageing Dev. 2000;113:61-70.

192. Zeng BY, Medhurst AD, Jackson M, Rose S, Jenner P. Proteasomal activity in brain differs between species and brain regions and changes with age. Mech Ageing Dev. 2005;126:760-6.

193. Floor E, Wetzel MG. Increased protein oxidation in human substantia nigra pars compacta in comparison with basal ganglia and prefrontal cortex measured with an improved dinitrophenylhydrazine assay. J Neurochem. 1998;70:268-75.

194. El-Khodor BF, Kholodilov NG, Yarygina O, Burke RE. The expression of mRNAs for the proteasome complex is developmentally regulated in the rat mesencephalon. Brain Res Dev Brain Res. 2001;129:47-56.

195. Conway KA, Rochet JC, Bieganski RM, Lansbury PT Jr. Kinetic stabilization of the alpha-synuclein protofibril by a dopamine-alpha-synuclein adduct. Science. 2001;294:1346-9.

196. Cappai R, Leck SL, Tew DJ, Williamson NA, Smith DP, Galatis D, Sharples RA, Curtain CC, Ali FE, Cherny RA, Culvenor JG, Bottomley SP, Masters CL, Barnham KJ, Hill AF. Dopamine promotes alpha-synuclein aggregation into SDS-resistant soluble oligomers via a distinct folding pathway. FASEB J. 2005;19:1377-9.

197. Gibb WR, Lees AJ. The relevance of the Lewy body to the pathogenesis of idiopathic Parkinson's disease. J Neurol Neurosurg Psychiatry. 1988;51:745-52.

198. Thrower JS, Hoffman L, Rechsteiner M, Pickart CM. Recognition of the polyubiquitin proteolytic signal. EMBO J. 2000;19:94-102.

199. Pickart CM. Ubiquitin enters the new millennium. Mol Cell. 2001;8:499-504.

200. Lam YA, Lawson TG, Velayutham M, Zweier JL, Pickart CM. A proteasomal ATPase subunit recognizes the polyubiquitin degradation signal. Nature. 2002;416:763-7.

5

Orthostatic Hypotension and Autonomic Dysfunction

Louise Allan

Address correspondence to Dr. Louise Allan, Institute for Ageing and Health, University of Newcastle upon Tyne, Newcastle General Hospital, Westgate Road, Newcastle upon Tyne, NE4 6BE, UK.
E-mail: louise.allan@ncl.ac.uk

OUTLINE

Introduction
      Orthostatic Hypotension
      Falls
Assessment of Autonomic Function
      Ewing Battery
      Heart Rate Variability
      Cardiac Scintigraphy
      Mechanisms of Autonomic Dysfunction in DLB and PDD
References

INTRODUCTION

Patients with autonomic failure experience disabling postural dizziness, syncope, falls, constipation, and incontinence[1]. The generalized deficit in cholinergic function in dementia with Lewy bodies (DLB) and Parkinson's disease dementia (PDD) would be expected to lead to autonomic dysfunction[2], and the Braak staging of Parkinson's disease[3] emphasizes early involvement of the brain stem, including the dorsal vagal nucleus. Autonomic failure has long been associated with Parkinson's disease[4–6], which many investigators now believe to be part of a spectrum of "Lewy Body Disorders" including Parkinson's disease, PDD, DLB, and pure autonomic failure[7]. If this is the case, one might expect that DLB as well as PDD would also be associated with autonomic failure.

It has been suggested that early symptoms of orthostatic dizziness, urinary incontinence, and constipation, in addition to syncope and falls, are suggestive of DLB or PDD rather than Alzheimer's disease, and may be attributable to underlying autonomic dysfunction. This view is consistent with previous evidence that there is a high prevalence of autonomic symptoms in Parkinson's disease[8] and other α-synucleinopathies, including DLB[9]. Retrospective case series have reported orthostatic dizziness and syncope as presenting or early symptoms of DLB[10,11,13,14], and syncope and falls have been included as supporting features in the diagnostic criteria for DLB[12]. In a retrospective examination of DLB patients, urinary incontinence and constipation were the most commonly documented autonomic symptoms[13], and one prospective study suggested that urinary incontinence occurs earlier in DLB than in Alzheimer's disease[14].

Autonomic symptoms have recently been reported to be more common in people with DLB and PDD than in people with other dementias. The report highlighted the clinical importance of autonomic symptoms in dementia and Parkinson's disease, particularly fatigue, postural dizziness, urinary symptoms, and constipation. Autonomic symptoms were strongly associated with reduced physical activity, depression, and impaired activities of daily living in these individuals[15]. Dependency in activities of daily living is a predictor of nursing home placement[16] and mortality in patients with dementia[17]. Autonomic symptoms were also significantly associated with greater impairment of quality of life, probably mediated by the reduction in activities of daily living, which have been shown to have a major impact on quality of life indices in a number of studies.

Physical inactivity is known to impair autonomic function and it is possible that the reduction in physical activity in patients with PDD and DLB causes secondary reduction in autonomic function. However, neuropathological studies demonstrating the presence of Lewy bodies in the autonomic nervous system of PDD and DLB patients suggest that autonomic dysfunction is not entirely due to physical inactivity[18–21]. It is possible that the patient's desire to engage in both physical activity and activities of daily living is reduced by both gait and balance impairment due to motor disorder, and the knowledge that such activities will be accompanied by unpleasant consequences, such as postural dizziness, thereby exacerbating the decline in functional ability and leading to a reduction in physical activity and, thus, further autonomic dysfunction.

Orthostatic Hypotension

Orthostatic hypotension (OH) is a common problem among older people living in the community, with a prevalence between 4 and 33% depending on the assessment methodology used and differences in population characteristics[22]. OH has been shown to be more common in all late-onset dementias than in healthy older people in several prospective studies (see Table 1), and can be contributed to by a number of other factors in addition to autonomic dysfunction.

The frequency of OH is possibly even higher in DLB than in other dementias, with recent data suggesting that the severity of the orthostatic drop, a more sustained orthostatic response, and a greater severity of associated symptoms were particularly characteristic of DLB[4]. The effects of autonomic dysfunction are important to clarify for several reasons. First, it might be used as an instrument to diagnose and differentiate different types of dementia from each other. Second,

Table 1. Summary of Studies Examining the Prevalence of OH in Dementia

Paper	Healthy Controls	AD	VAD	FTD	DLB	PD/PDD	Length of Stand
[25]	9%	0%					5 min
[26]						58% PD	
[27]	60%	33%					Not stated
[28]		39%	52%	46%			10 min
[29]		41%					Not stated
[30]		32%			40%		2 min
[31]		29%			93%		10 min
[32]					63%		Not stated
[33]						45% (included PD and PDD)	Not stated
[34]						14% (de novo PD)	3 min
[35]						47% (included PD and PDD)	2 min
[36]	13%	34%	34%		52%	49% PDD	3 min

it is important to recognize a low blood pressure in patients with dementia, as many of the drugs used to treat dementia have blood pressure–lowering properties and specific interventions may be necessary to improve related symptoms and reduce the risk of falls. Furthermore, there are additional potential adverse sequelae to hypotensive episodes. The drop in systolic blood pressure (SBP) induced by carotid sinus stimulation has been found to correlate with the severity of deep white matter lesions from microvascular disease, and patients with DLB have a greater and more prolonged slowing of heart rate and drop in SBP in response to carotid sinus massage than those with Alzheimer's disease or controls[23,24]. This indicates a possible connection between brain pathology and blood pressure derangement, which may exacerbate cognitive decline.

Falls

In older people, falls can have serious adverse outcomes, such as fractures, frequently leading to institutionalization and death[37,38].

Falls are a common feature of dementia and patients with dementia recover less well after a fall than those without dementia, and falls are a significant cause of increased morbidity, institutionalization, and mortality in these individuals[39]. There is a need to identify symptomatic dysautonomia in dementia in order to ensure appropriate management and reduce the risk of falls. Autonomic symptoms can be associated with falls and syncope, although the proportion of falls in these individuals attributable to autonomic dysfunction needs to be clarified by further research. Improved awareness of autonomic symptoms in dementia may, however, lead to earlier diagnosis of significant autonomic failure and appropriate intervention, which may have the potential to reduce falls and syncope. In older people without cognitive impairment, simple measures (such as adequate hydration, support hosiery, and pharmacological treatments, such as fludrocortisone and midodrine) can be used to manage symptomatic OH as part of a multifactorial intervention to reduce the risk of falls. There has only been one previous study of similar multifactorial interventions in people with dementia, but this was in a severely impaired group presenting to an emergency department following a fall[40]. Trials of multifactorial fall interventions for people with mild to moderate dementia are still required.

ASSESSMENT OF AUTONOMIC FUNCTION

Ewing Battery

The best-established clinical evaluation of autonomic function is incorporated within the Ewing battery, which includes three tests of parasympathetic function (heart rate responses to deep breathing, to standing, and to Valsalva maneuver) and three tests of sympathetic function (blood pressure responses to standing, to Valsalva maneuver, and to isometric exercise). These types of data can then be summarized by classifying each bedside autonomic test as normal or abnormal, based on percentiles, to produce an overall rating of autonomic function such as that illustrated in Table 2. OH, particularly if sustained, also suggests autonomic dysfunction, but can be multifactorial and is influenced by numerous cardiovascular medications.

Table 2. Ewing Battery

Normal	All tests normal or one borderline
Early	One of the three heart rate tests abnormal or two borderline
Definite	Two or more of the heart rate tests abnormal
Severe	Two or more of the heart rate tests abnormal plus one or both of the blood pressure tests abnormal or both borderline
Atypical	Any other combination

Recent work has highlighted specific abnormalities in these assessments in DLB and PDD (summarized in Table 3)[36].

Table 3. Ewing Battery in Patients with DLB and PDD in Comparison with Healthy Controls (Significant Results in Bold $*p < 0.05$, $**p < 0.01$)

Diagnosis	CONTROL	DLB	PDD
Mean change in heart rate during deep breathing	8.15	4.28**	3.98**
Mean 30:15 ratio (heart rate response to standing)	1.15	1.10*	1.05**
Mean Valsalva Ratio	1.43	1.28*	1.15**
Mean fall in SBP on standing (mm Hg)	26.6	43.2*	48.2**
Mean change in SBP during phase IV of Valsalva maneuver (mm Hg)	16.5	7.92	0.792**
Mean change in diastolic blood pressure on isometric exercise (mm Hg)	17.2	15.4	4.67**

Heart Rate Variability

Alterations in heart rate variability (HRV) are also indicative of autonomic failure and can be evaluated from further processing of a digitally recorded electrocardiogram (ECG). Power spectral analysis of the edited recording enables spectral bands in the very low (<0.04 Hz), low (0.04–0.15 Hz), and high (0.15–0.40 Hz) frequency ranges, and total spectral power (<0.40 Hz) to be obtained[16]. Sympathovagal balance can then be examined to determine the low to high frequency ratio. This technique has particular advantages for assessing autonomic function in people with dementia, where comprehension of and compliance with clinical autonomic function tests are not always possible. Several prior studies have investigated HRV in Alzheimer's disease[3,29], one identifying an absolute reduction in total spectral power and each frequency band, but the other failing to replicate these observations. Although there are few studies in PDD and DLB, recent work suggests that total spectral power, low frequency power, and high frequency power are reduced in PDD and DLB patients in comparison to people with Alzheimer's disease[36].

Cardiac Scintigraphy

The origin of sympathetic dysfunction in Lewy body diseases has been thought to be due mainly to peripheral sympathetic denervation[41]. Scintigraphy with [I-123]metaiodobenzyl guanidine ([I-123]MIBG)[31] enables the quantification of this postganglionic sympathetic cardiac innervation and the technique has been demonstrated to be useful in the identification of cardiac sympathetic denervation in Parkinson's disease and DLB[31,42]. The technique has been suggested to have high sensitivity and specificity in the differential diagnosis of DLB from Alzheimer's disease, and is included within the new operationalized clinical criteria for DLB as a "suggestive feature"[12].

Mechanisms of Autonomic Dysfunction in DLB and PDD

Lewy body pathology can also be found in medullary regions that control preganglionic sympathetic neurons, but with relative preservation of catecholaminergic neuronal populations[18], although previous work has suggested that medullary pathology is closely related to autonomic dysfunction in multisystem atrophy[43]. My own work[36] suggests that sympathetic dysfunction is present in PDD and DLB, but less marked in DLB patients. This raises the possibility that there may be a differential susceptibility and order of involvement of central and peripheral autonomic neurons to Lewy body pathology in DLB and PDD. This needs to be addressed in comparative neuropathological studies of the autonomic nervous system, but highlights a potentially important pathological difference between the two conditions.

As acetylcholine is essential for parasympathetic and preganglionic sympathetic neurotransmission, cholinergic dysfunction has also been discussed as a potential cause of autonomic failure in dementia patients[44] and may be particularly important in PDD and DLB, where cholinergic deficits are especially pronounced and where the disease pathology involves the dorsal vagal nucleus. In this context, it will be important to determine the impact of cholinesterase inhibitor therapy in dementia patients with autonomic impairment. Preliminary reports do suggest an adverse effect of donepezil on autonomic function, leading to carotid sinus hypersensitivity and falls in some individuals[45]. The general impact of cholinesterase inhibitors on autonomic function is difficult to determine from the existing clinical trial literature given the selected nature of the patient populations, but will be important to establish for clinical practice where patients are frailer and more likely to have autonomic symptoms.

REFERENCES

1. Low PA, Opfer-Gehrking TL, McPhee BR, et al. Prospective evaluation of clinical characteristics of orthostatic hypotension. Mayo Clin Proc. 1995;70(7):617-22.

2. Perry EK, Smith CJ, Court JA, Perry RH. Cholinergic nicotinic and muscarinic receptors in dementia of Alzheimer, Parkinson and Lewy body types. J Neural Transm Park Dis Dement Sect. 1990;2(3):149-58.

3. Braak H, Del Tredici K, Rub U, et al. Staging of brain pathology related to sporadic Parkinson's disease. Neurobiol Aging. 2003;24(2):197-211.

4. Martignoni E, Pacchetti C, Godi L, et al. Autonomic disorders in Parkinson's disease. J Neural Transm Suppl. 1995;45:11-9.

5. Koike Y, Takahashi A. Autonomic dysfunction in Parkinson's disease. Eur Neurol. 1997;38 Suppl 2:8-12.

6. Chaudhuri KR. Autonomic dysfunction in movement disorders. Curr Opin Neurol. 2001;14(4):505-11.

7. Hishikawa N, Hashizume Y, Yoshida M, Sobue G. Clinical and neuropathological correlates of Lewy body disease. Acta Neuropathol (Berl). 2003;105(4):341-50.

8. Korchounov A, Kessler KR, Yakhno NN, et al. Determinants of autonomic dysfunction in idiopathic Parkinson's disease. J Neurol. 2005;252(12):1530-6.

9. McKeith IG. Clinical Lewy body syndromes. Ann N Y Acad Sci. 2000;920:1-8.

10. Wenning GK, Scherfler C, Granata R, et al. Time course of symptomatic orthostatic hypotension and urinary incontinence in patients with postmortem confirmed parkinsonian syndromes: a clinicopathological study. J Neurol Neurosurg Psychiatry. 1999;67(5):620-3.

11. Thaisetthawatkul P, Boeve BF, Benarroch EE, et al. Autonomic dysfunction in dementia with Lewy bodies. Neurology. 2004;62(10):1804-9.

12. McKeith IG, Dickson DW, Lowe J, et al. Diagnosis and management of dementia with Lewy bodies: third report of the DLB consortium. Neurology. 2005;65:1863-72.

13. Del Ser T, Hachinski V, Merskey H, Munoz DG. Clinical and pathologic features of two groups of patients with dementia with Lewy bodies: effect of coexisting Alzheimer-type lesion load. Alzheimer Dis Assoc Disord. 2001;15(1):31-44.

14. Del-Ser T, Munoz DG, Hachinski V. Temporal pattern of cognitive decline and incontinence is different in Alzheimer's disease and diffuse Lewy body disease. Neurology. 1996;46(3):682-6.

15. Allan L, McKeith I, Ballard C, Kenny RA. The prevalence of autonomic symptoms in dementia and their association with physical activity, activities of daily living and quality of life. Dement Geriatr Cogn Disord. 2006;22(3):230-7.

16. Yaffe K, Fox P, Newcomer R, et al. Patient and caregiver characteristics and nursing home placement in patients with dementia. JAMA. 2002;287(16):2090-7.

17. Cohen-Mansfield J, Marx MS, Lipson S, Werner P. Predictors of mortality in nursing home residents. J Clin Epidemiol. 1999;52(4):273-80.

18. Benarroch EE, Schmeichel AM, Low PA, et al. Involvement of medullary regions controlling sympathetic output in Lewy body disease. Brain. 2005;128(Pt 2):338-44.

19. Orimo S, Amino T, Itoh Y, et al. Cardiac sympathetic denervation precedes neuronal loss in the sympathetic ganglia in Lewy body disease. Acta Neuropathol (Berl). 2005;109(6):583-8.

20. Okada Y, Ito Y, Aida J, et al. Lewy bodies in the sinoatrial nodal ganglion: clinicopathological studies. Pathol Int. 2004;54(9):682-7.

21. Jellinger KA. Lewy body-related alpha-synucleinopathy in the aged human brain. J Neural Transm. 2004;111(10-11):1219-35.

22. Hale WA, Chambliss ML. Should primary care patients be screened for orthostatic hypotension? J Fam Pract. 1999;48(7):547-52.

23.   Ballard C, O'Brien J, Barber B, et al. Neurocardiovascular instability, hypotensive episodes, and MRI lesions in neurodegenerative dementia. Ann N Y Acad Sci. 2000;903:442-5.

24.   Kenny RA, Shaw FE, O'Brien JT, et al. Carotid sinus syndrome is common in dementia with Lewy bodies and correlates with deep white matter lesions. J Neurol Neurosurg Psychiatry. 2004;75(7):966-71.

25.   Idiaquez J, Rios L, Sandoval E. Postprandial hypotension in Alzheimer's disease. Clin Auton Res. 1997;7(3):119-20.

26.   Senard JM, Rai S, Lapeyre-Mestre M, et al. Prevalence of orthostatic hypotension in Parkinson's disease. J Neurol Neurosurg Psychiatry. 1997;63(5):584-9.

27.   Siennicki-Lantz A, Lilja B, Elmstahl S. Orthostatic hypotension in Alzheimer's disease: result or cause of brain dysfunction? Aging (Milano). 1999;11(3):155-60.

28.   Passant U, Warkentin S, Gustafson L. Orthostatic hypotension and low blood pressure in organic dementia: a study of prevalence and related clinical characteristics. Int J Geriatr Psychiatry. 1997;12(3):395-403.

29.   Lebert F, Mouly C, Pasquier F. Tolerance to tacrine, arterial hypotension and leuko-araiosis in Alzheimer's disease. Age Ageing. 1998;27(5):654.

30.   Ballard C, Shaw F, McKeith I, Kenny R. High prevalence of neurovascular instability in neurodegenerative dementias. Neurology. 1998;51(6):1760-2.

31.   Yoshita M, Taki J, Yamada M. A clinical role for [(123)I]MIBG myocardial scintigraphy in the distinction between dementia of the Alzheimer's-type and dementia with Lewy bodies. J Neurol Neurosurg Psychiatry. 2001;71(5):583-8.

32.   Watanabe H, Ieda T, Katayama T, et al. Cardiac (123)I-meta-iodobenzylguanidine (MIBG) uptake in dementia with Lewy bodies: comparison with Alzheimer's disease. J Neurol Neurosurg Psychiatry. 2001;70(6):781-3.

33.   Wood BH, Bilclough JA, Bowron A, Walker RW. Incidence and prediction of falls in Parkinson's disease: a prospective multidisciplinary study. J Neurol Neurosurg Psychiatry. 2002;72(6):721-5.

34.   Bonuccelli U, Lucetti C, Del Dotto P, et al. Orthostatic hypotension in de novo Parkinson disease. Arch Neurol. 2003;60(10):1400-4.

35.   Allcock LM, Ullyart K, Kenny RA, Burn DJ. Frequency of orthostatic hypotension in a community based cohort of patients with

Parkinson's disease. J Neurol Neurosurg Psychiatry. 2004;75(10):1470-1.

36. Allan LM, Ballard CG, Allen J, et al. Autonomic dysfunction in dementia. J Neurol Neurosurg Psychiatry. 2006 [Epub ahead of print]

37. Tinetti ME, Inouye SK, Gill TM, Doucette JT. Shared risk factors for falls, incontinence, and functional dependence. Unifying the approach to geriatric syndromes. JAMA. 1995;273(17):1348-53.

38. Tinetti ME, Williams CS. Falls, injuries due to falls, and the risk of admission to a nursing home. N Engl J Med. 1997;337(18):1279-84.

39. Shaw FE. Falls in cognitive impairment and dementia. Clin Geriatr Med. 2002;18(2):159-73.

40. Shaw FE, Bond J, Richardson DA, et al. Multifactorial intervention after a fall in older people with cognitive impairment and dementia presenting to the accident and emergency department: randomised controlled trial. BMJ. 2003;326(7380):73.

41. Goldstein DS, Holmes CS, Dendi R, et al. Orthostatic hypotension from sympathetic denervation in Parkinson's disease. Neurology. 2002;58(8):1247-55.

42. Taki J, Yoshita M, Yamada M, Tonami N. Significance of 123I-MIBG scintigraphy as a pathophysiological indicator in the assessment of Parkinson's disease and related disorders: it can be a specific marker for Lewy body disease. Ann Nucl Med. 2004;18(6):453-61.

43. Benarroch EE, Smithson IL, Low PA, Parisi JE. Depletion of catecholaminergic neurons of the rostral ventrolateral medulla in multiple systems atrophy with autonomic failure. Ann Neurol. 1998;43(2):156-63.

44. Kenny RA, Allan, LM. Autonomic dysfunction in Dementia with Lewy bodies. In Dementia with Lewy Bodies and Parkinson's Disease Dementia. Edited by O'Brien, J. et al. London: Taylor and Francis; 2005:107-27.

45. McLaren AT, Allen J, Murray A, et al. Cardiovascular effects of donepezil in patients with dementia. Dement Geriatr Cogn Disord. 2003;15(4):183-8.

6

Relationship of Parkinson's Disease with Dementia and Dementia with Lewy Bodies

Dag Aarsland[1] and Clive Ballard[2]

[1]University Hospital, Stavanger, Norway;
[2]King's College London.

Address correspondence to Dr. Dag Aarsland Centre for Clinical Neuroscience Research, University Hospital, Stavanger and School of Medicine, University of Bergen, Bergen, Norway.
E-mail: daa@sir.no

OUTLINE

Introduction
Comparative Morphological and Neurochemical Studies
    Neuropathology
    Neurochemistry
Comparative Studies of Clinical Features in PDD and DLB
    Cognitive Deficits
    Psychiatric Symptoms
    Parkinsonism
    Disease Course
Imaging
Clinicopathological Dimensions Rather than Categories
References

INTRODUCTION

Dementias with Lewy bodies (DLB) and Parkinson's disease dementia (PDD) are characterized by parkinsonism and a dementia syndrome typically dominated by attentional, visuospatial, and executive dysfunction, and relatively preserved memory. Additional key symptoms are visual hallucinations, cognitive fluctuations, and sleep disturbances, such as excessive daytime sleepiness and REM sleep behavioral disorder (a parasomnia manifested by vivid, often frightening, dreams associated with simple or complex behavior during REM sleep)[1].

The distinction between DLB and PDD as operationally defined within the standardized clinical criteria depends entirely on the duration of parkinsonism prior to dementia. An arbitrary cut-off of 1 year has been chosen and, thus, PDD is diagnosed if dementia occurs more than 1 year after onset of parkinsonism, whereas dementia prior to or within 1 year after onset of parkinsonism is classified as DLB. There is currently little evidence on which to base the relationship between DLB and PDD, and several key conceptual questions remain unresolved; for example, are these conditions distinct or part of the same spectrum? If they are distinct conditions, is the arbitrary 1-year rule a meaningful distinction between clinical entities with different clinical presentations? Addressing these issues is critical to take forward our understanding of this spectrum of conditions; establishing biological markers, determining prognostic indicators, and most importantly, in designing appropriate intervention studies and developing treatment paradigms across the dementias associated with cortical Lewy bodies.

Direct comparative studies are the design to explore the relationship between DLB and PDD, but methodological limitations preclude clear conclusions. Critical issues include the selection of subjects (i.e., whether community based or hospital based); whether subjects were matched for severity of dementia, sample size, sensitivity, and other psychometric properties of the tests used to characterize the patients; and diagnostic criteria and methods of diagnosis (e.g., diagnosis based on autopsy, prospective clinical assessment, or retrospective chart review). Many studies comparing neuropathology or neurochemistry in Parkinson's disease and DLB did not specify whether Parkinson's disease patients had dementia or not. Since these two groups differ markedly in this regard, the interpretation of results from most of these studies is difficult. Nevertheless, although major differences between DLB and PDD have not been reported, some differences in clinical phenotype and brain changes have been reported. These will be highlighted, and we will aim to synthesize similarities and differences, and propose a model that highlights brain-behavior relationship rather than categorical entities.

COMPARATIVE MORPHOLOGICAL AND NEUROCHEMICAL STUDIES

Neuropathology

DLB and PDD cannot be differentiated by neuropathology alone. Both syndromes share limited atrophy compared to Alzheimer's disease. Medial temporal lobe structures are abnormal in both DLB and PDD, although the severity of hippocampal atrophy is less marked than that seen in Alzheimer's disease. Both Lewy body disorders have significant, but similar, atrophy and pathology in the amygdala[2].

Limbic and cortical Lewy bodies are the main substrate of the clinical dementia syndrome in DLB and PDD[3–5]. Alzheimer-type pathology is sparse, in particular neurofibrillary tangles, but may nevertheless influence the clinical phenotype in DLB[6,7]. In many cortical regions, the amount of Lewy body pathology does not differentiate DLB from PDD or Parkinson's disease[4,5], although higher Lewy body densities in parahippocampal and inferior temporal cortices in DLB compared to PDD have been reported[8]. Such differences may underlie the subtle clinical differences between the two syndromes. For example, the density of temporal lobe Lewy bodies in DLB correlates with the early occurrence of the characteristic well-formed visual hallucinations. In contrast, increasing Lewy body densities in limbic and frontal cortices in PDD correlate with the severity of dementia[9,10]. This dichotomy of regional Lewy body pathology suggests that the disease processes driving DLB and PDD differ.

The density of amyloid plaques was found to be higher in DLB than in PDD, with the density of Aβ-positive plaques in DLB equivalent to that found in Alzheimer's disease. While the amount of Aβ deposition and cortical Lewy bodies correlated with dementia severity in DLB, this does not seem to be the case in PDD[4]. However, in a recent study, such differences were not found[5]. In DLB, but not Parkinson's disease, there is a marked Lewy body neurodegeneration in the striatum, although Parkinson's disease patients with dementia had binding levels intermediate between Parkinson's disease and DLB[11]. One possible explanation for this finding is an interaction between amyloid plaques and α-synuclein aggregation. Overall, these findings support the concept of a continuum of Lewy body disease rather than two distinct diseases.

Neurochemistry

Neurochemically, both syndromes are characterized by cholinergic and nigrostriatal dopaminergic deficits. However, the severity and regional pattern of dopamine loss differ. More marked nigral cell loss occurs in PDD[5,12], but compensatory pre- and postsynaptic up-regulation of dopamine receptors occurs in PDD, but not in DLB[12]. Thus, the net striatal dopamine output may be quite similar, corresponding with the rather similar profile and severity of parkinsonism in the two syndromes.

Cortical cholinergic deficits secondary to cell loss of forebrain nuclei are pronounced in DLB and PDD[13]. These deficits are even more severe than in Alzheimer's disease[14], and are associated with decreased performance on tests of attentional and executive functioning[15]. In addition, cholinergic deficits have been reported in selected thalamic nuclei in PDD[16]. There is evidence linking cholinergic changes, in particular nicotinic modulation of thalamocortical circuitry, with the disturbed consciousness in patients with DLB[17].

The impact on cortical cholinergic receptors is similar in PDD and DLB with increased muscarinic binding and a considerable reduction in nicotinic binding[18]. Differential cholinergic changes have been reported in DLB and PDD. In the insular cortex, the cholinergic deficits were more marked in PDD than DLB[19]. In DLB, but probably not PDD, there is a correlation between visual hallucinations and cholinergic deficits in the temporal cortex[20].

Importantly, there is pronounced clinical heterogeneity *within* the two syndromes, and preliminary evidence indicates that the differences within PDD may be even more substantial than between PDD and DLB. For example, some Parkinson's disease patients may develop dementia early in course, whereas others remain cognitively intact or develop dementia late in course[21]. Studying the relationship between the time from onset of Parkinson's disease to dementia, we found that those with early dementia (i.e., less than 10 years after onset of Parkinson's disease) had similar morphological and neurochemical changes as those with DLB, whereas Parkinson's disease patients with late-onset dementia had less morphological cortical pathology (Lewy bodies, amyloid plaques, neurofibrillary tangles), but more severe cholinergic deficit in temporal cortex[22].

COMPARATIVE STUDIES OF CLINICAL FEATURES IN PDD AND DLB

Cognitive Deficits

The overall profile of cognitive deficits is quite similar in the two syndromes, with both PDD and DLB patients exhibiting significantly more marked executive and attention deficit, fluctuating attention, and less severe memory deficits than those patients with Alzheimer's disease[13]. Some studies have reported more pronounced executive dysfunction in DLB than PDD, in particular in mild dementia[23,24]. In addition, a recent study of prepulse inhibition, a paradigm that enables the study of basic attention processes independent of task understanding and deliberate participation, demonstrated more pronounced impairment in DLB than PDD[25]. Although studies based on group means provide important information, comparison of group means may disguise heterogeneity within the groups. Indeed, recent evidence has demonstrated that in Parkinson's disease and in PDD, subgroups with different cognitive profiles exist. The majority of patients have an executive-visuospatial–dominant profile, whereas others have a memory-dominant profile[26,27]. Similarly, some DLB patients, probably those with more abundant Alzheimer-type changes, may lack the characteristic Lewy body profile.

Psychiatric Symptoms

The psychiatric profile in DLB and PDD is characteristic and similar; visual hallucinations being the most common and most typical psychiatric symptom[7,28,29]. Although a similar pattern of symptoms and similar psychotic phenotype have been reported in PDD and DLB[30], visual hallucinations, misidentification, and delusions are more common in DLB than in PDD, possibly due to morphological and/or neurochemical differences as reported above. The characteristic psychiatric profile in DLB is less pronounced in those with more severe Alzheimer-type lesions[6,7].

Parkinsonism

It has frequently been suggested, based largely on anecdote, that parkinsonism is less severe in patients with DLB than in those with Parkinson's disease. Of note, a proportion of DLB patients do not have parkinsonism, but in those who have, severity and profile of parkinsonism is rather similar to the findings in PDD, and parkinsonism is a key factor that explains the functional impairment in DLB[31]. In the most detailed comparative study of parkinsonism to date, Burn et al. found that DLB patients had less severe parkinsonism than those with PDD, but a similar severity of motor deficits compared to Parkinson's disease patients without dementia[32]. Postural instability and gait difficulties, predominantly mediated by nondopaminergic lesions, were more pronounced in DLB and PDD patients than in Parkinson's disease patients without dementia, whereas the opposite was found for tremor. In a prospective study, those who had postural instability and gait difficulties–dominant

Parkinson's disease at baseline, or developed this after having tremor-dominant Parkinson's disease initially, had a much higher risk of dementia compared to those who maintained a tremor-type Parkinson's disease[33].

Disease Course

Only one study has directly compared the course of clinical features in PDD and DLB. This study reported that DLB and PDD patients had a similar rate of decline of cognition and motor symptoms over 2 years[34]. There are some indications that the course of disease is more severe in PDD and DLB than in Alzheimer's disease, although this has not yet been substantiated statistically. Similarly, whether mortality and risk of nursing home admission is higher in DLB and PDD than in Alzheimer's disease is not clear.

IMAGING

In the first study comparing magnetic resonance imaging in DLB and PDD patients, cortical atrophy in both groups differed from Alzheimer's disease patients and normal controls, but no significant differences were found between DLB and PDD using voxel-based morphometry[35]. Similarly, whereas DLB and PDD patients had medial temporal lobe atrophy compared to healthy subjects, but less severe than Alzheimer's disease patients, there were no differences between DLB and PDD[36]. However, preliminary results from our group, using similar methodology, suggest that DLB patients have more widespread cortical atrophy than PDD patients, even with a similar degree of overall dementia.

Functional imaging studies have revealed characteristic patterns in patients with DLB and PDD compared to those with nondemented Parkinson's disease, Alzheimer's disease, and normal controls. Most characteristic is the visualization by means of several different tracers of the nigrostriatal dopamine system, demonstrating striatal abnormalities in Parkinson's disease and DLB patients, compared to Alzheimer's disease patients and healthy controls[37,38]. A slightly different pattern in DLB and PDD has been shown: Parkinson's disease and PDD patients show more left-right asymmetry and a more posterior striatal degeneration compared to PDD patients[37,38]. A similar rate of decline of striatal binding in PDD and DLB has been shown[39].

Studies of the cerebral cortical blood flow have demonstrated characteristic patterns in DLB as well as PDD. Cerebral perfusion deficits are confined mainly to either parietal or occipital regions, or both, in DLB as compared to Alzheimer's disease, whereas reductions in all cortical lobes have been reported in PDD[40]. Comparative studies have reported slightly different regional patterns of cerebral blood flow in DLB and PDD. In one study, DLB patients had a more markedly reduced blood flow in the frontal lobe[41]. In another study, the pattern was similar, but DLB patients had a more pronounced overall reduction of cerebral blood flow than PDD patients[42]. Longitudinal studies have reported progressive reduction of frontal lobe blood flow in Parkinson's disease[43], but no significant change in PDD[44]. Few studies have explored the associations between regional functional changes and specific clinical features. A recent longitudinal study reported correlations between increase in perfusion in midline posterior cingulate and decrease in hallucination severity, and between fluctuations of consciousness and increased thalamic and decreased inferior occipital perfusion[45].

CLINICOPATHOLOGICAL DIMENSIONS RATHER THAN CATEGORIES

There are many similarities in the type and frequency of clinical features diagnostic for DLB and PDD, although the severity of executive dysfunction and frequency of visual hallucinations and delusions are more pronounced in DLB than in PDD. However, methodological limitations preclude firm conclusions regarding the similarities or differences between the two syndromes. In addition, marked differences exist *within* the two syndromes. Some DLB patients have a very characteristic clinical profile with visuospatial and executive dysfunction, visual hallucinations, and parkinsonism, whereas others have a clinical profile more similar to that seen in patients with Alzheimer's disease. Similarly, some Parkinson's disease patients develop dementia early in course, whereas others remain nondemented or develop it late in course. Some develop visual hallucinations or severe psychosis, whereas others do not show these symptoms despite large doses of dopaminergic antiparkinson drugs.

Although major brain differences between PDD and DLB do not exist, subtle neurochemical and pathological differences are likely to subserve the clinical differences. A more pronounced executive dysfunction in DLB may relate to the loss of the hippocampal projection to the frontal lobe in DLB, but not Parkinson's disease, and more severe Lewy body pathology in the inferior temporal lobe may relate to the higher frequency of visual hallucinations in DLB. The differential pattern of parkinsonian features in Parkinson's disease and DLB is in accordance with the differential striatal changes, with changes in PDD patients being intermediate between those found in DLB and Parkinson's disease patients. Similarly, within the two syndromes, the severity of Alzheimer-type changes is associated with a less-classical DLB phenotype. In PDD, those who develop dementia early have more pronounced cortical morphological changes. More studies are needed to address the relationship between these syndromes by understanding the relationship of the underlying pathological and neurochemical substrates to the clinical profile and course of PDD and DLB.

The available data strongly support a "continuum" model, and indicate that any arbitrary clinical distinction between DLB and PDD does not reflect the pattern of cortical neuropathological and neurochemical changes. As the majority of previous research has focused on the distinction between DLB and PDD, future studies should combine DLB and PDD patients, and aim to disentangle empirically based subgroups within the continuum of Lewy body dementia. This will enable further work to focus on the pathological and neurochemical processes underpinning the clinical phenotypes across the full spectrum, with the potential to understand prognosis and to develop and evaluate new targeted treatment approaches.

REFERENCES

1. McKeith IG, Dickson DW, Lowe J, et al. Diagnosis and management of dementia with Lewy bodies: third report of the DLB consortium. Neurology. 2005;65:1863-72.

2. Cordato NJ, Halliday GM, Harding AJ, Hely MA, Morris JG. Regional brain atrophy in progressive supranuclear palsy and Lewy body disease. Ann Neurol. 2000;47:718-28.

3. Aarsland D, Perry R, Brown A, Larsen JP, Ballard C. Neuropathology of dementia in Parkinson's disease: a prospective, community-based study. Ann Neurol. 2005;58:773-6.

4. Harding AJ, Halliday GM. Cortical Lewy body pathology in the diagnosis of dementia. Acta Neuropathol (Berl). 2001;102:355-63.

5. Tsuboi Y, Dickson DW. Dementia with Lewy bodies and Parkinson's disease with dementia: are they different? Parkinsonism Relat Disord. 2005;11 Suppl 1:S47-51.

6. Merdes AR, Hansen LA, Jeste DV, et al. Influence of Alzheimer pathology on clinical diagnostic accuracy in dementia with Lewy bodies. Neurology. 2003;60:1586-90.

7. Ballard CG, Jacoby R, Del Ser T, et al. Neuropathological substrates of psychiatric symptoms in prospectively studied patients with autopsy-confirmed dementia with Lewy bodies. Am J Psychiatry. 2004;161:843-9.

8. Harding AJ, Broe GA, Halliday GM. Visual hallucinations in Lewy body disease relate to Lewy bodies in the temporal lobe. Brain. 2002;125:391-403.

9. Samuel W, Galasko D, Masliah E, Hansen LA. Neocortical Lewy body counts correlate with dementia in the Lewy body variant of Alzheimer's disease. J Neuropathol Exp Neurol. 1996;55:44-52.

10. Kovari E, Gold G, Herrmann FR, et al. Lewy body densities in the entorhinal and anterior cingulate cortex predict cognitive deficits in Parkinson's disease. Acta Neuropathol (Berl). 2003;106:83-8.

11. Duda JE, Giasson BI, Mabon ME, Lee VM, Trojanowski JQ. Novel antibodies to synuclein show abundant striatal pathology in Lewy body diseases. Ann Neurol. 2002;52:205-10.

12. Piggott MA, Marshall EF, Thomas N, et al. Striatal dopaminergic markers in dementia with Lewy bodies, Alzheimer's and Parkinson's diseases: rostrocaudal distribution. Brain. 1999;122(Pt 8):1449-68.

13. Aarsland D, Ballard CG, Halliday G. Are Parkinson's disease with dementia and dementia with Lewy bodies the same entity? J Geriatr Psychiatry Neurol. 2004;17:137-45.

14. Bohnen NI, Kaufer DI, Ivanco LS, et al. Cortical cholinergic function is more severely affected in parkinsonian dementia than in Alzheimer disease: an in vivo positron emission tomographic study. Arch Neurol. 2003;60:1745-8.

15. Bohnen NI, Kaufer DI, Hendrickson R, et al. Cognitive correlates of cortical cholinergic denervation in Parkinson's disease and parkinsonian dementia. J Neurol. 2006;253:242-7.

16. Ziabreva I, Ballard CG, Aarsland D, et al. Lewy body disease: thalamic cholinergic activity related to dementia and parkinsonism. Neurobiol Aging. 2006;27:433-8.

17. Pimlott SL, Piggott M, Ballard C, et al. Thalamic nicotinic receptors implicated in disturbed consciousness in dementia with Lewy bodies. Neurobiol Dis. 2006;21:50-6.

18. Aarsland D, Mosimann UP, McKeith IG. Role of cholinesterase inhibitors in Parkinson's disease and dementia with Lewy bodies. J Geriatr Psychiatry Neurol. 2004;17:164-71.

19. Pimlott SL, Piggott M, Owens J, et al. Nicotinic acetylcholine receptor distribution in Alzheimer's disease, dementia with Lewy bodies, Parkinson's disease, and vascular dementia: in vitro binding study using 5-[(125)i]-a-85380. Neuropsychopharmacology. 2004;29:108-16.

20. Ballard C, Piggott M, Johnson M, et al. Delusions associated with elevated muscarinic binding in dementia with Lewy bodies. Ann Neurol. 2000;48:868-76.

21. Aarsland D, Kvaløy JT, Andersen K, Larsen JP, Tang MX, Lolk A, Kragh-Sørensen P, Marder K. The effect of age of onset of PD on risk of dementia. J Neurol. in press.

22. Ballard C, Ziabreva I, Perry R, Larsen JP, O'Brien JO, McKeith I, Perry E, Aarsland D. Difference in neuropathologic characteristics across the Lewy body dementia spectrum. Neurology. 2007;67:1931-4

23. Aarsland D, Litvan I, Salmon D, Galasko D, Wentzel-Larsen T, Larsen JP. Performance on the dementia rating scale in Parkinson's disease with dementia and dementia with Lewy bodies: comparison with progressive supranuclear palsy and Alzheimer's disease. J Neurol Neurosurg Psychiatry. 2003;74:1215-20.

24. Downes JJ, Priestley NM, Doran M, Ferran J, Ghadiali E, Cooper P. Intellectual, mnemonic, and frontal functions in dementia with Lewy bodies: a comparison with early and advanced Parkinson's disease. Behav Neurol. 1998;11:173-83.

25. Perriol MP, Dujardin K, Derambure P, et al. Disturbance of sensory filtering in dementia with Lewy bodies: comparison with Parkinson's

disease dementia and Alzheimer's disease. J Neurol Neurosurg Psychiatry. 2005;76:106-8.

26. Foltynie T, Brayne CE, Robbins TW, Barker RA. The cognitive ability of an incident cohort of Parkinson's patients in the UK. The CamPaIGN study. Brain. 2004;127:550-60.

27. Janvin CC, Larsen JP, Aarsland D, Hugdahl K. Subtypes of mild cognitive impairment in Parkinson's disease: progression to dementia. Mov Disord. 2006;21(9):1343-9.

28. Aarsland D, Bronnick K, Ehrt U, et al. Neuropsychiatric symptoms in patients with Parkinson's disease and dementia: frequency, profile and associated care giver stress. J Neurol Neurosurg Psychiatry. 2007;78(1):36-42.

29. Aarsland D, Cummings JL. Psychiatric aspects of Parkinson's disease, Parkinson's disease with dementia, and dementia with Lewy bodies. J Geriatr Psychiatry Neurol. 2004;17:111.

30. Mosimann UP, Rowan EN, Partington CE, et al. Characteristics of visual hallucinations in Parkinson disease dementia and dementia with Lewy bodies. Am J Geriatr Psychiatry. 2006;14:153-60.

31. McKeith IG, Rowan E, Askew K, et al. More severe functional impairment in dementia with Lewy bodies than Alzheimer disease is related to extrapyramidal motor dysfunction. Am J Geriatr Psychiatry. 2006;14:582-8.

32. Burn DJ, Rowan EN, Minett T, et al. Extrapyramidal features in Parkinson's disease with and without dementia and dementia with Lewy bodies: a cross-sectional comparative study. Mov Disord. 2003;18:884-9.

33. Alves G, Larsen JP, Emre M, Wentzel-Larsen T, Aarsland D. Changes in motor subtype and risk for incident dementia in Parkinson's disease. Mov Disord. 2006;21(8):1123-30.

34. Burn DJ, Rowan EN, Allan LM, Molloy S, O'Brien JT, McKeith IG. Motor subtype and cognitive decline in Parkinson's disease, Parkinson's disease with dementia, and dementia with Lewy bodies. J Neurol Neurosurg Psychiatry. 2006;77:585-9.

35. Burton EJ, McKeith IG, Burn DJ, Williams ED, O'Brien JT. Cerebral atrophy in Parkinson's disease with and without dementia: a comparison with Alzheimer's disease, dementia with Lewy bodies and controls. Brain. 2004;127:791-800.

36. Tam CW, Burton EJ, McKeith IG, Burn DJ, O'Brien JT. Temporal lobe atrophy on MRI in Parkinson disease with dementia: a comparison with Alzheimer disease and dementia with Lewy bodies. Neurology. 2005;64:861-5.

37. O'Brien JT, Colloby S, Fenwick J, et al. Dopamine transporter loss visualized with FP-CIT SPECT in the differential diagnosis of dementia with Lewy bodies. Arch Neurol. 2004;61:919-25.

38. Walker Z, Costa DC, Walker RW, et al. Striatal dopamine transporter in dementia with Lewy bodies and Parkinson disease: a comparison. Neurology. 2004;62:1568-72.

39. Colloby SJ, Williams ED, Burn DJ, Lloyd JJ, McKeith IG, O'Brien JT. Progression of dopaminergic degeneration in dementia with Lewy bodies and Parkinson's disease with and without dementia assessed using 123I-FP-CIT SPECT. Eur J Nucl Med Mol Imaging. 2005;32:1176-85.

40. Colloby S, O'Brien J. Functional imaging in Parkinson's disease and dementia with Lewy bodies. J Geriatr Psychiatry Neurol. 2004;17:158-63.

41. Kasama S, Tachibana H, Kawabata K, Yoshikawa H. Cerebral blood flow in Parkinson's disease, dementia with Lewy bodies, and Alzheimer's disease according to three-dimensional stereotactic surface projection imaging. Dement Geriatr Cogn Disord. 2005;19:266-75.

42. Mito Y, Yoshida K, Yabe I, et al. Brain 3D-SSP SPECT analysis in dementia with Lewy bodies, Parkinson's disease with and without dementia, and Alzheimer's disease. Clin Neurol Neurosurg. 2005;107:396-403.

43. Firbank MJ, Molloy S, McKeith IG, Burn DJ, O'Brien JT. Longitudinal change in 99mTcHMPAO cerebral perfusion SPECT in Parkinson's disease over one year. J Neurol Neurosurg Psychiatry. 2005;76:1448-51.

44. Firbank MJ, Burn DJ, McKeith IG, O'Brien JT. Longitudinal study of cerebral blood flow SPECT in Parkinson's disease with dementia, and dementia with Lewy bodies. Int J Geriatr Psychiatry. 2005;20:776-82.

45. O'Brien JT, Firbank MJ, Mosimann UP, Burn DJ, McKeith IG. Change in perfusion, hallucinations and fluctuations in consciousness in dementia with Lewy bodies. Psychiatry Res. 2005;139:79-88.

7

Clinical Management of Dementia with Lewy Bodies and Parkinson's Disease Dementia: Key Issues

Clive Ballard[1] and Dag Aarsland[2]

[1]Wolfson Centre for Age-Related Diseases; Institute of Psychiatry, King's College London, UK;
[2]University Hospital, Stavanger, Norway.

Address correspondence to Dr. Clive Ballard, Wolfson Centre for Age-Related Diseases, Wolfson Wing, Hodgkin Building, Guy's Campus, King's College London, London, SE1 1UL, UK.
E-mail: Clive.ballard@kcl.ac.uk

OUTLINE

Introduction
Accurate Diagnosis
General Pharmacologic Treatments for DLB and PDD
Other General Pharmacologic Treatments
Neuropsychiatric Symptoms
    Mood Disorders
        Depression
        Anxiety
        Apathy
    Parkinsonism
    Falls and Dysautonomia
Conclusion
References

INTRODUCTION

Dementia with Lewy bodies (DLB) and Parkinson's disease dementia (PDD) are characterized by progressive cognitive impairment, with prominent attentional and visuospatial dysfunction, severe neuropsychiatric symptoms, fluctuating cognition, parkinsonism, autonomic dysfunction, sleep disorders, and a vulnerability to falls and related injuries[1].

This complex combination of distressing symptoms creates a number of difficult dilemmas for optimal management. The evidence base informing the clinical management of DLB is still limited, requiring recommendations to be based on a combination of this evidence, together with clinical experience of managing these patients. Given the complex and difficult issues facing the clinician, management preferably should be coordinated within a specialist center[2].

ACCURATE DIAGNOSIS

A first and essential step towards clinical management is to make an accurate diagnosis. The previous consensus criteria for the diagnosis of DLB[3] have been shown to have good specificity, but limited sensitivity, in clinicopathological studies, with several studies achieving sensitivities below 50%[4]. Clearly, this is a major problem, as a substantial number of patients with DLB are not being identified even when the operationalized diagnostic criteria are being applied and, under diagnosis, it is likely to be even more problematic in routine practice. In addition to the general treatment benefits of making the correct diagnosis, this could potentially expose a large number of patients to the risk of severe neuroleptic sensitivity reactions[5–7]. The main reason for the difficulties in applying the operationalized clinical criteria has been the challenge of identifying fluctuating cognition, with several studies suggesting that agreement between clinicians is barely better than chance[8,9]. Utilizing the rating scales that have now been validated[10–12] and assessing variability in reaction time on formal assessments of attention should, however, enable more accurate assessment of fluctuation. Other potential difficulties include patients with a combination of cerebrovascular and Lewy body pathology, and assessment of spontaneous parkinsonism in people who take neuroleptics or who have severe dementia.

The revised operationalized criteria[1] may assist with the general diagnostic accuracy. The presence of REM sleep behavior disorder and the results of investigations, such as DAT and MIBG scans, now form part of the diagnostic criteria, which should help to improve sensitivity, although this has not yet been evaluated systematically. Given the particular challenges of managing patients with DLB, the best advice is probably to consider DLB as the most likely clinical diagnosis if there are any suggestive features.

The diagnosis of PDD poses other difficulties. As more than 90% of patients who develop dementia meet operationalized criteria for DLB and cortical Lewy body pathology is the main substrate of dementia in these individuals[13], differential diagnosis between different dementias is not problematic in the majority of situations. However, many people with Parkinson's disease have subtle cognitive deficits and rigorous longitudinal evaluation is advisable as part of the clinical follow-up to enable the diagnosis of dementia to be made as early as possible.

Given the complex combination of symptoms in people with DLB and PDD, it is helpful to think about the different treatment targets. Ultimately, the goal is to identify therapies that fundamentally impact on the disease process. There is some emerging evidence that cholinesterase inhibitors (ChEIs) may reduce the accumulation or impact of concurrent amyloid pathology[14], and a number of other potentially exciting avenues are being explored, such as the relationship between proteasome function and α-synuclein pathology[15]. However, these remain research questions at the moment and clinical management, therefore, needs to focus on key symptoms. DLB and PDD are both progressive neurodegenerative dementias associated with global cognitive deterioration, and impairment of self-care and other activities of daily living. As with all dementias, improving cognition and stabilizing self-care skills are major treatment goals. However, in DLB and PDD, prominent neuropsychiatric symptoms, parkinsonism, falls, autonomic dysfunction, or sleep disorders may be the most important symptoms for a particular individual. It is helpful, therefore, to document the symptoms that require assessment and treatment in a therapeutic plan based on a problem list of key symptoms, prioritized in order of importance to the patient. Caregiver opinion about the impact of particular symptoms should also be inquired about, particularly since some disturbances, e.g., sleep or behavioral, may have the most impact on them. Before any pharmacological intervention, it is helpful to explain that improvements in one symptom domain may lead to deterioration in others, and that slow and careful titration of drug dose may help to reduce this. Frequent monitoring for response to treatment and adverse effects of medications is recommended.

GENERAL PHARMACOLOGIC TREATMENTS FOR DLB AND PDD

The main evidence base for treating cognitive symptoms pertains to the use of acetyl ChEIs. The first trial was a small, open-label study of seven patients with PDD treated with tacrine, who experienced improvement in cognition (Mini-Mental State Examination [MMSE] score) and visual hallucinations. The trial suggested that, contrary to previous concerns, parkinsonian symptoms actually improved. Although the potential utility of tacrine is limited by the high risk of hepatotoxicity, the trial was extremely important in highlighting the potential value of ChEI therapy[16]. Aarsland et al.[27] have summarized the literature and highlighted 14 small studies that focus on ChEI treatment in patients with Parkinson's disease with an open or randomized cross-over design, including a total of 144 patients and trials with tacrine, donepezil, rivastigmine, and galantamine between 1996 and 2003. Overall MMSE scores improved by approximately two points and more than 90% of patients had an improvement in their visual hallucinations. Although the overall balance of the literature did not support[16] the suggestion of an improvement in motor symptoms, only a very modest proportion of individuals experienced a worsening of parkinsonism. The only large, parallel, group, randomized, controlled trial (RCT) of a ChEI in PDD, published in

2004[17], confirmed the impression from the previous preliminary studies and demonstrated that rivastigmine was significantly better than placebo over 24 weeks of treatment, in 541 patients with PDD (allocated 2:1 rivastigmine:placebo). Over the treatment period, the rivastigmine-treated patients had a one-point advantage on the MMSE, an almost three-point advantage on the ADAS-COG, and significant benefits on more specialized assessment of attention and executive function. There were also significant two-point advantages for rivastigmine-treated patients on the ADCS activity of daily living scale and the neuropsychiatric inventory. Although there was no overall significant worsening of parkinsonism, there was a significant increase of tremor as a reported adverse event in the rivastigmine-treated patients and, as expected, the participants receiving rivastigmine were more likely to experience nausea (29 versus 11%) and vomiting (16.5 versus 2%). There was no difference in falls, with 75% of participants able to tolerate rivastigmine for the duration of the study. Mortality rates were significantly lower in the rivastigmine-treated patients (1.1 versus 3.9%).

A similar evolution of studies was seen for DLB with initial small case series[18,19], indicating that two-thirds of patients experienced benefit from ChEI treatment, especially with respect to neuropsychiatric symptoms, and several reports[20] highlight improvements in fluctuating confusion. In general, this literature supports the conclusions of the treatment studies in PDD, indicating that parkinsonian symptoms only worsened in a minority of individuals, although in one of the reports[18], three of the nine patients experienced a worsening of their parkinsonism. Again, this literature emphasized the need for a randomized, controlled, clinical trial, culminating in a multicenter, placebo-controlled trial[21] of 120 DLB patients treated with rivastigmine (mean dose 7 mg) or placebo for 2 weeks. The primary outcome measure was 30% improvement in a four-item subscore (delusions, hallucinations, apathy, depression), which was attained by 63% of people treated with rivastigmine and 30% of people treated with placebo, a significant difference on the observed case analysis. On the total neuropsychiatric inventory (NPI), there was a nonsignificant three-point advantage to the rivastigmine-treated patients. It should be emphasized, however, that this difference was not evident at the 12-week assessment point, and the benefit appeared to emerge between 12 and 20 weeks. The impact on specific psychiatric symptoms and fluctuating cognition has been less well studied. Significant improvements were also seen in attentional performance, with a nonsignificant, one-point advantage to the rivastigmine-treated patients on the MMSE. The reports of adverse events were similar to those in the subsequent PDD trial.

The overall literature is extremely encouraging, with evidence from two large RCTs that were supported by an extensive case series literature, indicating that rivastigmine is significantly better than placebo for the treatment of cognitive deficits and neuropsychiatric symptoms; with evidence from the PDD study[17] that there are also significant advantages for activities of daily living.

Rivastigmine is well tolerated, with no significant exacerbation of parkinsonism, although nausea and vomiting can be a problem. In addition, detrusor instability is common in DLB patients, can occur early in the course of the illness[22], and may be exacerbated by ChEIs. The case series literature suggests that donepezil is also an effective treatment for DLB and PDD, and individual studies also indicate benefits with tacrine and galantamine. While this suggests that the treatment efficacy is a ChEI class effect overall, the only robust RCT evidence is for rivastigmine. In the absence of direct comparative studies, it is difficult to make any firm conclusions about the relative efficacy of the different ChEIs. One large 2-year RCT comparing rivastigmine and donepezil for the treatment of Alzheimer's disease did suggest a modest advantage for rivastigmine in the subgroup of patients who met criteria for possible DLB, but the diagnostic status of these patients is very unclear. The profile of adverse events has not been directly compared in DLB or PDD patients either, although the literature in Alzheimer's disease probably indicates that, on balance, nausea and vomiting may be more frequent in people treated with rivastigmine, although this may be largely a consequence of too rapid a titration in some of the studies. One small cross-over study with donepezil in a combined cohort of DLB and Alzheimer's disease patients did indicate a significant exacerbation of syncope and carotid sinus hypersensitivity (CSH) and related falls in donepezil-treated patients[23]. This is a very real clinical concern given the high frequency of CSH and other aspects of autonomic dysfunction in DLB and PDD patients, but it is unclear whether the propensity to exacerbate these problems differs between the different ChEIs. An ECG, assessment of autonomic function and postural hypotension, and a good clinical history to evaluate syncope should probably be completed before instigating treatment, and any emergent symptoms/features of autonomic dysfunction should be monitored carefully during therapy.

As ChEIs exacerbate rather than help urinary incontinence, other management approaches may be necessary. Anticholinergics, such as oxybutinin, often used to treat urinary frequency, can cross the blood brain barrier and may worsen cognitive function, so non-pharmacological approaches are preferable.

Several reports have attempted to evaluate predictors of treatment response within the RCT. The presence of visual hallucinations or more severe attentional impairments, probably both markers of more severe cholinergic deficits, are both associated with preferential treatment response[24].

OTHER GENERAL PHARMACOLOGIC TREATMENTS

There is limited or no evidence regarding the use of other candidate therapies, such as memantine, vitamin E, or selegeline, and clinical trials of these treatments are an important research priority.

NEUROPSYCHIATRIC SYMPTOMS

Visual hallucinations, delusions, and accompanying agitation are frequent in DLB and PDD, each occurring in 60% of DLB or PDD patients cross-sectionally[25]. When assessing the treatment of these symptoms, it is critical to determine whether there is any medical comorbidity, review potentially contributing medications, assess relevant visual impairments, and determine the severity of the symptoms and the level of distress caused to the person and their carergiver. In particular, attention should be paid to the potential contributing role of antiparkinsonian medications, and dose reduction or even discontinuation of some antiparkinsonian medications may be indicated.

Nonpharmacological interventions have been shown to ameliorate neuropsychiatric symptoms effectively in people with dementia, but have not yet been evaluated systematically in DLB. Approaches vary in complexity from optimizing the care and support package, and promoting good communication and person-centered care, to specific tailored interventions involving the patient, caregiver, and/or environment[26]. If symptoms are not causing enormous distress, nonpharmacological treatments should probably be the intervention of first choice, although ChEIs prescribed as a more generic pharmacotherapy may confer additional benefit.

When specific pharmacological intervention is required to treat neuropsychiatric symptoms in DLB or PDD, the main options are ChEIs or atypical, antipsychotic medications. Open-label and placebo-controlled studies have demonstrated the effectiveness of all three generally available ChEIs on visual hallucinations, delusions, and associated agitation in DLB and PDD (for review see Aarsland et al.[27]), with a reduction in both symptom frequency and intensity, which appears to be mediated at least in part by improved attentional function[24]. The RCTs in DLB and PDD have compared rivastigmine to placebo, and show a general improvement in neuropsychiatric symptoms, but the specific impact on visual hallucinations has not been reported and the time course to improvement appears to be 3–6 months. Although there is some disparity between the case series and the RCT data, a trial of a ChEI will give general benefits, is well tolerated, and is the pharmacological treatment of first choice. There are no comparative data between the ChEIs in PDD or DLB, although given the higher level of evidence, rivastigmine is probably the treatment of choice. Beneficial effects of ChEIs may be sustained for at least 2 years of treatment[28] and sudden withdrawal may precipitate marked deterioration in neuropsychiatric symptoms[29]. If symptoms are particularly severe and distressing, the time frame of response to ChEI therapy may be too slow.

The use of atypical neuroleptics creates a much more difficult clinical dilemma because of the general potential for adverse events and the specific risk of severe neuroleptic sensitivity reactions in DLB and PDD patients[5–7]. Widely reported general side effects of neuroleptics include parkinsonism, drowsiness, dystonia, and abnormal involuntary movements (tardive dyskinesia) associated with long-term treatment; with many agents also causing anticholinergic side effects, including delirium. In people with Alzheimer's disease, recent data have also highlighted serious risks, including cerebrovascular adverse events[30] and increased mortality[31]. Combining data from the placebo-controlled trials in people with Alzheimer's disease, risperidone is associated with a significant threefold increased risk of serious cerebrovascular adverse events (defined within the studies as including stroke, transient ischemic attacks, and a range of other vascular events including syncope) compared to placebo[30]. Summary data supplied by Eli Lilly and Company Ltd suggest a similar increase in the incidence of cerebrovascular adverse events in the placebo-controlled trials of olanzapine in Alzheimer's disease (olanzapine 1.3% versus placebo 0.4%) and cautions have also been issued pertaining to aripiprazole. Schneider et al.[31] reviewed the evidence from 15 of these trials, confirming a significant 1.5-fold increase in mortality, but finding no difference between specific agents. A very recent report indicates that the mortality risk may be even higher with typical neuroleptics[32]. These risks may be acceptable for the short-term treatment of severe and distressing neuropsychiatric symptoms, but are a major concern over longer periods of therapy. In DLB and PDD, there is the additional specific problem of severe neuroleptic sensitivity reactions. McKeith et al.[5] reported that 50% of neuroleptic-treated patients with DLB experienced severe drug sensitivity, with symptoms that included marked extrapyramidal features, confusion, autonomic instability, falls, and accelerated mortality. An accumulating literature of case reports and case series, as well as subsequent larger and more systematic series, shows that severe sensitivity reactions occur with a wide range of typical and atypical antipsychotics, including clozapine, in DLB and the related condition of PDD patients[6,7]. Failure of neuroleptic prescriptions to up-regulate dopamine D2 receptors has been highlighted as a major factor contributing to severe neuroleptic sensitivity[33]. However, the largest and most systematic study suggested that the highest frequency of severe neuroleptic sensitivity reactions occurred in olanzapine-treated patients[7], raising the possibility that antimuscarinic properties may also be important. Clinically, severe neuroleptic sensitivity reactions are a major concern, as they can occur after only a few[6] or even single doses of neuroleptics[34]. There is clear evidence from RCTs in Alzheimer's disease patients with behavioral and psychiatric symptoms that atypical neuroleptics are an effective treatment for the short-term (6–12 weeks) treatment of aggression, but with more marginal benefits for psychosis and other symptoms of agitation[30,31]. There are no placebo-controlled trials in DLB patients, but one reanalysis of an Alzheimer's disease trial in which a small proportion of participants met clinical criteria for possible DLB, and several other small open trials, indicate some improvement of neuropsychiatric symptoms with olanzapine[35] and quetiapine[36] treatment. Several larger open trials in people with Parkinson's disease suggest improvement in psychotic symptoms[37]. Our view is that balancing the risks of therapy with atypical antipsychotics and the limited specific evidence of benefit in DLB and PDD, atypical antipsychotics should only be used for extremely severe neuropsychiatric symptoms, where there is extreme distress or risk to the patient or others. If therapy is instigated, it should be undertaken with extremely close monitoring over the first 2 weeks, especially the first 2–3 days, so that any early indications of severe neuroleptic sensitivity reactions or other major adverse events can be identified and treatment discontinued as soon as possible.

In Alzheimer's disease, there is some evidence from cross-over studies and RCTs that anticonvulsants, such as carbamazepine and sodium valproate, and antidpepresants, such as trazadone and citalopram, may improve some neuropsychiatric symptoms[30]. The evidence is limited, however, and mainly indicates potential benefit for agitation symptoms rather than psychotic symptoms. There are no studies of these agents in people with DLB or PDD, and the safety of these treatment approaches has not been established in these individuals. The risk of falls, for example, may be a serious concern. Emerging data from Alzheimer's disease trials also suggest that memantine may confer benefit in the treatment of neuropsychiatric symptoms, although there have been several case reports of increased confusion in people with DLB who were treated with memantine and the potential utility of memantine therapy in DLB/PDD patients needs to be evaluated more systematically.

In a number of circumstances, the problematic situation may arise where people experience ongoing and distressing visual hallucinations or other neuropsychiatric symptoms that have not responded to ChEI treatment or nonpharmacological interventions. Although difficult, providing the appropriate support to enable people to manage and cope with the situation effectively is still probably a better option for most people than the potential risks of atypical antipsychotics.

Mood Disorders

Depression

Depression is very common in both DLB and PDD, and there have been no systematic studies of its management. At the present time, SSRI and SNRIs are probably preferred pharmacological treatments, although studies of SSRIs in Parkinson's disease without dementia have been disappointing. Tricylic antidepressants and those with anticholinergic properties should be avoided. Nonpharmacological interventions, such as activity programs, exercise, and cognitive behavior therapy, have been shown to be effective for the treatment of depression in Alzheimer's disease[38], but have not been evaluated for DLB.

Anxiety

Anxiety is also frequent and may be secondary to fluctuating confusion, psychotic features, or depression. Treating the underlying neuropsychiatric condition will often result in resolution. There is, however, no specific evidence base to provide information for the treatment of more severe or persistent symptoms. In studies of ChEIs in Alzheimer's disease, anxiety is often one of the symptoms that shows a preferential response[39]. Nonpharmacological interventions, similar to those utilized for depression, can be helpful and SSRIs may be worth considering. Benzodiazepines should probably be avoided because of the risks of worsening amnesia, decreased alertness, and impairment of motor function, with increased risk of falls.

Sleep disorders are also frequently seen in Lewy body disease and may be an early feature. They can be treated with clonazepam (0.25 mg) at bedtime, titrating slowly while monitoring for both efficacy and side effects[40]. ChEIs may also be helpful for disturbed sleep[41].

Apathy

Apathy, often associated with attentional and executive impairments, is a common feature that often adds to social and functional disability, and generally responds well to ChEIs[21].

Fluctuating cognition is often a prominent and distressing symptom, which adds to impairment on everyday activities and can create major practical problems for planning an appropriate care package. Several of the case series include patients whose fluctuating cognition improved with ChEI therapy, but the data are less clear-cut from the RCTs. In the McKeith et al.[21] study, for example, after adjusting for overall improvement in attentional performance, there was no specific improvement of fluctuation. Fluctuating cognition is an important treatment target that merits further research, but may be improved by ChEI treatment.

Parkinsonism

Parkinsonism, by definition, occurs in all people with PDD and probably develops in 80% of DLB patients over the course of their illness. The parkinsonian syndrome differs in only subtle ways between Parkinson's disease, PDD, and DLB, and progresses at a similar rate in the three disorders. Motor symptoms contribute to the disability experienced by DLB and PDD patients, and are associated with an increased risk of falls. Levodopa can be used for the motor disorder of both DLB and PDD, but doses should be titrated more carefully. Levodopa is generally well tolerated, but may increase confusion in a small proportion of patients[42]. Responsiveness to levodopa is more limited in both DLB and PDD patients, with significant improvement of parkinsonism seen in approximately half of PDD patients and a smaller proportion of individuals with DLB, although falls may be reduced even in some patients without optimal motor response. Caution should be exercised when adding other parkinsonian medications, including selegeline, amantadine, COMT inhibitors, and dopamine agonists, because of concerns about exacerbating confusion and psychosis (visual illusions, hallucinations, and delusions). Anticholinergics should also be avoided in both DLB and PDD. Cognition and psychosis should be monitored with standardized evaluations.

Motor disability including parkinsonism and postural instability may also be improved by physiotherapy and occupational therapy approaches. The unpredictable and fluctuating nature of cognitive and motor impairments can prove particularly frustrating to patients and caregivers. Education, discussion, and reassurance on how to deal with variable performance can help both parties to adopt a flexible approach, depending on the patient's functional level at a given time.

Falls and Dysautonomia

There is a high prevalence of falls in DLB and PDD, with a considerable risk of related injuries. Falls prevention is, therefore, a very important management consideration. Falls are very multifactorial in dementia patients, with a number of factors including parkinsonism (with or without postural instability), postural hypotension, muscle weakness, posture, confidence/anxiety, medication, and the environment all contributing. A broad approach is needed, which should include an evaluation of the patient's environment, the need for walking devices, physiotherapy for gait training, and other rehabilitation efforts. Blood pressure should be checked for orthostatic BP, and minimization of cardiac medications and benzodiazepines is recommended. Management of postural hypotension includes removal of medications that may be causative or contributory. If postural hypotension persists following medication adjustment, then additional pharmacological treatments might include fludrocortisone and midodrine. Syncope may be an important attributable cause of falls. If suggestive symptoms are apparent, a detailed cardiovascular assessment is recommended, including head-up tilt and carotid sinus massage in a specialist facility. Cardiac pacing may be beneficial in some of these patients. Protective underwear and careful attention to flooring may reduce the risk of serious injury of patients at high risk of falling.

CONCLUSION

DLB and PDD are progressive, neurodegenerative disorders characterized by cognitive impairment, parkinsonism, and prominent neuropsychiatric symptoms. The complex combination of symptoms can be distressing for the patients and problematic for the managing clinician. ChEIs give significant benefits with respect to cognition, function, and neuropsychiatric symptoms, but not all patients respond, and finding the optimal balance between the treatment of key symptoms, such as psychosis and parkinsonism, and the risk of adverse events is often a major challenge.

REFERENCES

1. McKeith IG, Dickson DW, Lowe J, et al. Consortium on DLB. Diagnosis and management of dementia with Lewy bodies: third report of the DLB Consortium. Neurology. 2005;65:1863-72.
2. Barber R, Panikkar A, McKeith IG. Dementia with Lewy bodies: diagnosis and management. Int J Geriatr Psychiatry. 2001;16:12-8.
3. McKeith IG, Galasko D, Kosaka K, et al. Consensus guidelines for the clinical and pathologic diagnosis of dementia with Lewy bodies (DLB): report of the consortium on DLB international workshop. Neurology. 1996;47:1113-24.

4.   McKeith IG, O'Brien JT, Ballard C. Diagnosing dementia with Lewy bodies. Lancet. 1999;354:1227-8.

5.   McKeith I, Fairbairn A, Perry R, et al. Neuroleptic sensitivity in patients with senile dementia of Lewy body type. BMJ. 1992;305:673-4.

6.   Ballard C, Grace J, McKeith I, et al. Neuroleptic sensitivity in dementia with Lewy bodies and Alzheimer's disease. Lancet. 1998;351:1032-3.

7.   Aarsland D, Perry R, Larsen JP, et al. Neuroleptic sensitivity in Parkinson's disease and parkinsonian dementias. J Clin Psychiatry. 2005;66:633-7.

8.   Mega MS, Masterman DL, Benson DF, et al. Dementia with Lewy bodies: reliability and validity of clinical and pathologic criteria. Neurology. 1996;47:1403-9.

9.   Litvan I, MacIntyre A, Goetz CG, et al. Accuracy of the clinical diagnoses of Lewy body disease, Parkinson disease, and dementia with Lewy bodies: a clinicopathologic study. Arch Neurol. 1998;55:969-78.

10.   Walker MP, Ayre GA, Cummings JL, et al. The Clinician Assessment of Fluctuation and the One Day Fluctuation Assessment Scale. Two methods to assess fluctuating confusion in dementia. Br J Psychiatry. 2000;177:252-6.

11.   Ferman TJ, Boeve BF, Ivnik RJ, et al. DLB fluctuations: specific features that reliably differentiate from AD and normal aging. Neurology. 2004;62:181-7.

12.   Doubleday EK, Snowden JS, Varma AR, et al. Qualitative performance characteristics differentiate dementia with Lewy bodies and Alzheimer's disease. J Neurol Neurosurg Psychiatry. 2002;72:602-7.

13.   Aarsland D, Perry R, Brown A, et al. Neuropathology of dementia in Parkinson's disease: a prospective, community-based study. Ann Neurol. 2005;58:773-6.

14.   Kimura M, Komatsu H, Ogura H, et al. Comparison of donepezil and memantine for protective effect against amyloid-beta(1-42) toxicity in rat septal neurons. Neurosci Lett. 2005;391:17-21.

15.   McNaught KS, Belizaire R, Jenner P, Olanow CW. Isacson O. Selective loss of 20S proteasome alpha-subunits in the substantia nigra pars compacta in Parkinson's disease. Neurosci Lett. 2002;326:155-8.

16.   Hutchinson M, Fazzini E. Cholinesterase inhibition in Parkinson's disease. J Neurol Neurosurg Psychiatry. 1996;61:324-5.

17. Emre M, Aarsland D, Albanese A, et al. Rivastigmine for dementia associated with Parkinson's disease. N Engl J Med. 2004;351:2509-18.

18. Shea C, MacKnight C, Rockwood K. Donepezil for treatment of dementia with Lewy bodies: a case series of nine patients. Int Psychogeriatr. 1998;10:229-38.

19. Aarsland D, Bronnick K, Karlsen K. Donepezil for dementia with Lewy bodies: a case study. Int J Geriatr Psychiatry. 1999;14:69-72.

20. Kaufer DI, Catt KE, Lopez OL, et al. Dementia with Lewy bodies: response of delirium-like features to donepezil. Neurology 1998;51:1512.

21. McKeith I, Del Ser T, Spano P, et al. Efficacy of rivastigmine in dementia with Lewy bodies: a randomised, double-blind, placebo-controlled international study. Lancet. 2000;356:2031-6.

22. Del-Ser TD, Munoz G, et al. Temporal pattern of cognitive decline and incontinence is different in Alzheimer's disease and diffuse Lewy body disease. Neurology. 1996;46:682-6.

23. McLaren AT, Allen J, Murray A, et al. Cardiovascular effects of donepezil in patients with dementia. Dement Geriatr Cogn Disord. 2003;15:183-8.

24. McKeith IG, Wesnes KA, et al. Hallucinations predict attentional improvements with rivastigmine in dementia with Lewy bodies. Dement Geriatr Cogn Disord. 2004;18:94-100.

25. Ballard C, Holmes C, McKeith I, et al. Psychiatric morbidity in dementia with Lewy bodies: a prospective clinical and neuropathological comparative study with Alzheimer's disease. Am J Psychiatry. 1999;156:1039-45.

26. McKeith I, Mintzer J, et al. Dementia with Lewy bodies. Lancet Neurol. 2004;3:19-28.

27. Aarsland D, Mosimann UP, et al. Role of cholinesterase inhibitors in Parkinson's disease and dementia with Lewy bodies. J Geriatr Psychiatry Neurol. 2004;17:164-71.

28. Grace J, Daniel S, et al. Long-term use of rivastigmine in patients with dementia with Lewy bodies: an open-label trial. Int Psychogeriatr. 2001;13:199-205.

29. Minett TSC, Thomas A, et al. What happens when donepezil is suddenly withdrawn? An open label trial in dementia with Lewy bodies and Parkinson's disease with dementia. Int J Geriatr Psychiatry. 2003;18:988-93.

30. Ballard C, Howard R. Neuroleptic drugs in dementia: benefits and harm. Nat Rev Neurosci. 2006;7:492-500.

31. Schneider LS, Dagerman K, Insel PS. Efficacy and adverse effects of atypical antipsychotics for dementia: meta-analysis of randomized, placebo-controlled trials. Am J Geriatr Psychiatry. 2006;14:191-210.

32. Wang PS, Schneeweiss S, Avorn J, et al. Risk of death in elderly users of conventional vs. atypical antipsychotic medications. N Engl J Med. 2005;353:2335-41.

33. Piggott MA, Perry EK, Marshall EF, et al. Nigrostriatal dopaminergic activities in dementia with Lewy bodies in relation to neuroleptic sensitivity: comparisons with Parkinson's disease. Biol Psychiatry. 1998;44:765-74.

34. Sadek J, Rockwood K. Coma with accidental single dose of an atypical neuroleptic in a patient with Lewy body dementia. Am J Geriatr Psychiatry. 2003;11:112-3.

35. Cummings JL, Street J, Masterman D, et al. Efficacy of olanzapine in the treatment of psychosis in dementia with Lewy bodies. Dement Geriatr Cogn Disord. 2002;13:67-73.

36. Baskys, A. Lewy body dementia: the litmus test for neuroleptic sensitivity and extrapyramidal symptoms. J Clin Psychiatry. 2004;65:16-22.

37. Factor SA, Feustel PJ, Friedman JH, et al. Longitudinal outcome of Parkinson's disease patients with psychosis. Neurology. 2003;60:1756-61.

38. Teri L, Gibbons LE, McCurry SM, et al. Exercise plus behavioral management in patients with Alzheimer disease: a randomized controlled trial. JAMA. 2003;290:2015-22.

39. Gauthier S, Feldman H, Hecker J, Vellas B, Ames D, Subbiah P, Whalen E, Emir B; Donepezil MSAD Study Investigators Group. Efficacy of donepezil on behavioral symptoms in patients with moderate to severe Alzheimer's disease. Int Psychogeriatr. 2002;14:389-404.

40. Boeve BF, Silber MH, et al. REM sleep behavior disorder in Parkinson's disease and dementia with Lewy bodies. J Geriatr Psychiatry Neurol. 2004;17:146-57.

41. Reading PJ, Luce AK, et al. Rivastigmine in the treatment of parkinsonian psychosis and cognitive impairment. Mov Disord. 2001;16:1171-4.

42. Molloy S, McKeith IG, O'Brien JT, et al. The role of levodopa in the management of dementia with Lewy bodies. J Neurol Neurosurg Psychiatry. 2005;6:1200-3.

Index

A

B

C

D

Synaptophysin
  immunoreactivity, 12
Synphilin-1 (SNCAIP), 34

T

γ-tubulin, 77

U

Ubiquitin Carboxyl-Terminal
  Hydrolase L1 (UCH-L1,
  PARK5), 30
Ubiquitin C-terminal L1
  (UCH-L1), 30, 65

Ubiquitin staining, 3
Ubiquitination/
  deubiquitination, 79
Ubiquitin-proteasome system
  (UPS), 28, 61
Unwanted proteins, 79
UPS function, 76

V

Vesicular glutamate (VGLUT)
  transporter-1, 17

Printed in the United States
87090LV00001BB/129-206/A